A Handbook of Veterinary Parasitology

Domestic Animals of North America

A
Handbook of
Veterinary Parasitology

Domestic Animals
of
North America

Henry J. Griffiths

Professor, Veterinary Pathobiology
University of Minnesota

UNIVERSITY OF MINNESOTA PRESS □ MINNEAPOLIS

Preface

The presentation of material in this handbook is based on the author's experience in teaching veterinary parasitology. The information, concerning only parasites occurring in North America, has been compiled from the work and writings of many in the field of parasitology. Books devoted to veterinary parasitology are limited in number, and until now the highly regarded text by Soulsby was the only work in English dealing with the protozoans, arthropods, and helminths of veterinary importance.

The intent of the handbook is to provide the veterinary practitioner, student, and animal technician with an easily used source of information regarding the more common parasites of domestic animals in North America. The manual is not intended to be a standard text or an exhaustive source of information on animal parasites. It is designed to be a concise reference work from which the user may quickly retrieve factual material as an aid in the identification and control of animal parasites.

The material is presented in a consistent format. The parasites are listed alphabetically by scientific name within phylum or class. The common name is provided if sufficiently descriptive. The name is followed by pertinent information about each parasite such as its habitat, distribution, life cycle, transmission, disease signs, pathogenicity, diagnosis, and control. Although very important, little emphasis has been placed on morphology and taxonomy. The practitioner, with little time to devote to taxonomy, bases most parasite identification on host association and key morphological characteristics that may be seen grossly. Because parasites vary considerably in size among species and because the host influences the size of the parasite, average size ranges for adults and eggs are provided.

In the brief discussions of control, management practices and treatments are considered, and some of the more commonly used anthelmintics and insecticides are mentioned. Discussion of chemotherapeutic agents is limited because of rapid developments in the area of chemotherapy and the continual appearance of new products on the market. It is the author's belief that losses caused by parasites can only by reduced by the practice of preventive medicine based on knowledge of the parasite's biology and the use of appropriate chemotherapeutic agents.

In Appendix A a few of the common procedures used in the diagnosis of parasitic infections are outlined. A table of the more common parasites of domestic animals arranged by host is provided in Appendix B. Parasites of each host are grouped by the anatomical system or host tissue in which they occur. This table should help the reader determine the names of parasites likely found in various tissues. Appendix C contains brief information about some commonly used chemotherapeutic agents mentioned in the handbook. The parasites are listed alphabetically by specific name under each host heading.

Where appropriate, selected references to textbooks or journals to which the practitioner may have access are listed at the end of the entry for each parasite. If further references are desired, the reader is referred to the *Index Catalogue of Medical and Veterinary Zoology*, U.S.D.A., and to *Helminthological Abstracts*, Commonwealth Agricultural Bureaux. Both are invaluable sources of information.

The author is much indebted to the J. B. Lippincott Company for granting permission to draw freely from a chapter he wrote in *Veterinary Necropsy Procedures*. Special thanks are due Mrs. Rosemary MacFarlane for the excellent typing of the manuscript.

Table of Contents

PART I
PROTOZOANS

Protozoans

PARASITE: *Babesia bigemina*

Disease: Babesiosis (bovine), Texas fever, red water fever, piroplasmosis.
Host: Cattle, deer.
Habitat: Erythrocyte.
Identification: Trophozoites usually pyriform, may be round or oval, characteristically in pairs. Size is 2-3 μ in diameter and 4-5 μ long.
Distribution and importance: Until eradication was a major cattle disease in the southern U.S. It is important to the U.S. because of possible introduction from Mexico.
Life cycle: The trophozoite stage occurs in the erythrocyte where it multiplies by binary fission, budding, or schizogony. Reproductive stages are liberated from the erythrocyte and invade additional cells. Large numbers of erythrocytes may be parasitized.
Transmission: In North America, the natural arthropod vector is *Boophilus annulatus*. In Central and South America the usual vector is *B. microplus*. Transovarian transmission may occur in the tick. Mechanical transmission may result from the use of dirty instruments.
Signs and pathogenicity: In young animals the disease is frequently asymptomatic. Calves less than 1 year old are seldom seriously affected. In the mature animal the incubation period is 1-2 weeks following exposure to infective ticks. First sign of the disease is a spectacular rise in body temperature, to 106-108°F., which may last several days. In acute cases death occurs 4-8 days after onset of clinical signs. In chronic cases, animals become thin and emaciated and then slowly recover. At the height of the fever, 75% of the erythrocytes may be destroyed resulting in profound anemia. Necropsy shows splenomegaly, hepatomegaly, distended gall bladder, and icterus and edema of the digestive tract mucosa.
Diagnosis: Confirmed by detection of characteristic forms of the parasite within the erythrocyte. A complement fixation test is helpful in animals with a low parasitemia.

Control: Infection can be prevented by tick control, that is, regular dipping or spraying with an appropriate acaricide. Young stock to 1 year old are quite resistant and may be immunized by injection of blood from carrier animals. Intravenous inoculation of trypan blue, acriflavine, subcutaneous inoculations of phenamidine, and intramuscular injections of Berenil are proved, effective therapeutic agents. Elimination of babesiosis in the United States was accomplished by the regular dipping of cattle and thorough inspection and dipping of animals imported from tick-infested areas.

Selected references:

Malherbe, W. D. 1956. The manifestations and diagnosis of *Babesia* infections. *Ann. N. Y. Acad. Sci.* 64:128-46.

Neitz, W. O. 1956. Classification, transmission, and biology of piroplasms of domestic animals. *Ann. N. Y. Acad. Sci.* 64:56-111.

Smith, T., and F. L. Kilborne. 1893. Investigations into the nature, causation and prevention of Texas or southern cattle fever. U.S.D.A., *Bur. An. Ind. Bull.* 1:1-301.

PARASITE: *Babesia caballi*

Disease: Babesiosis (equine).

Host: Horse, mule, donkey.

Habitat: Erythrocyte.

Identification: Trophozoites pyriform, round, or oval and 2-4 μ long; characteristically in pairs. The points of the trophozoites are usually at an acute angle to each other.

Distribution and importance: Southern Florida and several other southern states. This disease is potentially important but has been controlled and eliminated to date. More than 400 cases were reported between 1961 and 1969.

Life cycle: Similar to *B. bigemina*.

Transmission: By bite of infected tick. *Dermacentor nitens* is the host in Florida. Transmission of organism in the tick is transovarian as well as transstadial. *D. nitens* is also thought to be mechanically transmitted by biting insects.

Signs and pathogenicity: The incubation period is 6-10 days. The disease may be acute or chronic. General signs are persistent fever, anemia, and icterus. Mortality may be 10-50% and may occur 1-4 weeks after onset of clinical signs. Recovered animals may remain carriers for one to several years. Central nervous system disturbances manifested by such signs as restlessness, nervousness, and walking incoordinately in circles may be observed.

Diagnosis: Direct demonstration of the parasites in the erythrocytes of the peripheral blood. Make smear from first drop of blood obtained from the rim of the ear. The complement fixation test is also claimed to be reliable.

Control: Accomplished by tick control and the treatment of carrier animals. Appropriate acaricides are toxaphene spray or dip. Treatment of the ears and false nostril with lindane in cottonseed oil is effective. Babesiacides of choice are Diampron, Berenil, Phenamidine isethionate, Acaprine, and trypan blue.

Selected references:

Bryant, J. E., J. B. Anderson, and K. H. Willers. 1969. Control of equine piroplasmosis in Florida. *J. Am. Vet. Med. Assoc.* 154:1034-36.

Holbrook. H. A., A. J. Johnson, and P. A. Madden. 1968. Equine piroplasmosis: intraerythrocytic development of *Babesia cabelli* and *Babesia equi. Am. J. Vet. Res.* 29:297-303.

Sippel, W. L., D. E. Cooperider, J. H. Gainer, R. W. Allen, J. E. B. Mouw, and M. B. Teigland. 1962. Equine piroplasmosis in the United States. *J. Am. Vet. Med. Assoc.* 141:694-98.

Taylor, W. M., J. E. Bryant, J. B. Anderson, and K. H. Willers. 1969. Equine piroplasmosis in the United States—a review. *J. Am. Vet. Med. Assoc.* 155:915-19.

PARASITE: *Babesia canis (Piroplasma canis)*

Disease: Babesiasis (canine), malignant jaundice, biliary fever, canine piroplasmosis.

Host: Dog and wild carnivores.

Habitat: Erythrocyte.

Identification: Organism pyriform, 4-5 μ long. Usually 1 pair to a cell, occasionally several pairs are seen in 1 erythrocyte.

Distribution and importance: Enzootic in the southern regions of North America and of importance in specific localities.

Life cycle: Not completely understood. Multiple infections of the erythrocytes occur. Trophozoites in the erythrocytes multiply by binary fission or schizogony. Merozoites have been described from endothelial cells of the lung and kidney. In the tick, transmission may be transovarian and transstadial.

Transmission: Bite of the infected ticks *Rhipicephalus sanguineus* and, probably, *Dermacentor* spp.

Signs and pathogenicity: Infection varies from quite mild to severe with the strain of the organism. Young and old dogs become infected; less severe disease occurs in the former. Incubation period is 10-21 days in naturally infected animals. Usual signs are fever of 102-105°F., loss of condition, anemia, icterus, prostration, and death. In chronic forms of the disease signs are vague. The patient may be listless, weak, and emaciated and have intermittent fever. The manifestations of disease are quite variable.

Diagnosis: Demonstration of parasite in the erythrocyte, best accomplished by taking capillary smears from the margin of the ear. Exposure of a susceptible, splenectomized dog to infective blood is a reliable diagnostic tool especially in areas where the disease is not enzootic. On necropsy, impression smears of the lung, liver, or kidney should be examined.

Control: Tick control and treatment of infected individuals. Acriflavine and trypaflavine have both given good results. Phenamidine is less toxic and quite effective.

Selected references:

Dikmans, G. 1935. Canine babesiasis in the United States. *N. Amer. Vet.* 16:45-48.

Ewing, S. A., and R. G. Buckner. 1965. Manifestations of babesiosis, ehrlichiosis and combined infections in the dog. *Am. J. Vet. Res.* 26:815-28.

Rokey, N. W. 1961. Canine babesiosis—a case report. *J. Am. Vet. Med. Assoc.* 138: 635-38.

Shortt, H. E. 1973. *Babesia canis:* the life cycle and laboratory maintenance in its arthropod and mammalian hosts. *Intl. J. Parasitol.* 3:119-48.

PARASITE: *Babesia equi*

Disease: Babesiosis (equine).

Host: Horse, mule, donkey.

Habitat: Erythrocyte.

Identification: Trophozoites may be round, ameboid, or pyriform. Four organisms may be joined, giving the effect of a Maltese cross. Individual organisms are 2-3 μ long.

Distribution and importance: A few cases have been reported from southern regions of North America, but it is presumed the disease has been eradicated.

Life cycle: Generally similar to that of *B. bovis* except that the trophozoite in the erythrocyte divides into 4 daughter trophozoites.

Transmission: The tick vectors are numerous. The carrier of *B. equi* in the U.S. is unknown, *B. equi* will not develop in *Dermacentor nitens*.

Signs and pathogenicity: In natural infections, incubation period is 1-3 weeks. A fever of 103-106°F. is characteristic, with anemia, icterus, depression, weakness, and edema.

Diagnosis: Organism found in the blood early in the period of fever. The first few drops of blood taken from the rim of the ear are most likely to contain the organism. At necropsy, impression smears of spleen, liver, and kidney usually contain organisms. The complement fixation test is accurate and reliable.

Control: Tick control. Foals less than 1 year old have strong resistance. Recovered animals have great resistance to reinfection. The most effective therapeutic agent seems to be phenamidine isethionate.

Selected references:

Ristic, M., J. Oppermann, S. Sibinovic, and T. N. Phillips. 1964. Equine piroplasmosis—a mixed strain of *Piroplasma caballi* and *Piroplasma equi* isolated in Florida and studied by the fluorescent-antibody technique. *Am. J. Vet. Res.* 25:15-23.

Sippel, W. L., D. E. Cooperider, J. H. Gainer, R. W. Allen, J. E. B. Mouw, and M. B. Teigland. 1962. Equine piroplasmosis in the United States. *J. Am. Vet. Med. Assoc.* 141:694-98.

Taylor, W. M., J. E. Bryant, J. B. Anderson, and K. H. Willers. 1969. Equine piroplasmosis in the United States—a review. *J. Am. Vet. Med. Assoc.* 155:915-19.

Thompson, P. H. 1969. Ticks as vectors of equine piro-plasmosis. *J. Am. Vet. Med. Assoc.* 155:454-57.

PARASITE: *Balantidium coli* (ciliate)

Disease: Balantidiasis.

Host: Pig, man, and occasionally dog.

Habitat: Cecum and colon.

Identification: Variable in size. Trophozoites may be 150 μ long and 120 μ wide. The macronucleus is sausage- to kidney-shaped. Cysts are spherical or ovoid, 40-60 μ in diameter, with a slight greenish-yellow tinge. The trophozoite, covered with numerous rows of cilia, may be readily recognized by its size, characteristic macronucleus, and lively motility.

Distribution and importance: Very common in hogs and widely distributed; of minor importance.

Life cycle: Reproduction is by transverse binary fission. Resistant cysts are formed.

Transmission: By ingestion of cysts or trophozoites. The latter are probably only infective if ingested in freshly passed feces. Man is usually thought to acquire infection from hogs through contamination of foodstuffs or by otherwise accidentally ingesting contaminated pig feces.

Signs and pathogenicity: This ciliate is generally considered a commensal in the large intestine of pigs. In man and other primates the organism may be a pathogen. It is reported to be the cause of diarrhea or dysentery and to be associated with ulcertaion of the muscularis mucosa. Occasionally this protozoan may invade the intestinal mucosa of pigs and cause severe enteritis and ulceration.

Diagnosis: May be easily recognized by microscopic examination of the intestinal contents or by histologic examination of lesions.

Control: General sanitation and prevention of ingestion of cysts. Usually treatment of the pig is unnecessary. Oxytetracycline and chlortetracycline have proved valuable in the treatment of man and would probably be suitable for use in swine if necessary.

Selected references:

Bailey, W. S., and A. G. Williams. 1949. *Balantidium* infection in the dog. *J. Am. Vet. Med. Assoc.* 114:238.

Levine, N. D. 1973. *Protozoan parasites of domestic animals and man.* 2nd ed. Minneapolis: Burgess. Pp. 369-71.

PARASITE: *Besnoitia besnoiti* (now considered to be a coccidium)

Disease: Besnoitiasis (Globidiosis).

Host: A variety of domestic and wild ruminants and laboratory animals.

Habitat: Trophozoites in the blood are extracellular or in monocytes; also found in lymph nodes and lung tissue. Cysts develop in subcutaneous tissues, fascia, mucosae of the nose, trachea, and other locations.

Identification: The pseudocyst is without septa and contains banana- or crescent-shaped trophozoites. Pseudocysts are more or less spherical and may be 500 μ in diameter; trophozoites are 2-7 μ long.

Distribution and importance: Not commonly seen in North America. Species have been reported from horse, reindeer, deer mouse, and opossum.

Life cycle: Considered to be similar to that of *Sarcocystis*, but to date its status has not been completely clarified.

Transmission: Natural transmission of *B. besnoiti* thought to be by the bite of a bloodsucking fly, a tabanid. The mosquito and the stable fly may transmit the parasite. In some hosts transmission may also occur through ingestion of infective tissue. Artificial transmission may be accomplished by intravenous or other forms of parenteral injection of infective blood from animals showing the acute phase of the disease.

Signs and pathogenicity: Animals 6 months or older may be infected. After an incubation period of 6-10 days, there is a temperature rise of short duration, a photophobia develops, and the hair loses its luster. Edema may develop along the underside of the body. Following initial signs, skin lesions appear in about 4 weeks. Skin thickening and wrinkling occurs, and hair is lost. In the terminal stage there is a seborrhea sicca. Denuded areas are covered by a scurfy layer, the skin hardens and becomes elephantlike. In general, cutaneous besnoitiasis is characterized by painful swellings, thickening of the skin, loss of hair with areas of necrosis, and general debilitation. In light infections with minor hair loss the animals will return to normal. In chronic cases, recovery may require months or years. Mortality may be about 10%.

Diagnosis: Confirmed by finding the cysts and demonstrating by biopsy the crescent-shaped trophozoite.

Control: No preventive or treatment measures are known. Control of tabanids might be considered.

Selected references:

Bigalke, R. D. 1968. New concepts on the epidemiological features of bovine besnoitiosis as determined by laboratory and field investigations. *Onderstepoort J. Vet. Res.* 35:3-137.

Pols, J. W. 1960. Studies on bovine besnoitiosis with special reference to the aetiology. *Onderstepoort J. Vet. Res.* 28:265-356.

PARASITE: *Eimeria bovis, E. auburnensis, E. zurnii.* Of the dozen or more species of bovine coccidia, these seem to be the more important.

Disease: Intestinal coccidiosis (bovine).

Host: Cattle and other large ruminants.

Habitat: *E. bovis:* Asexual generation in the ileum and later in the cecum and colon. *E. auburnensis:* In the middle and lower small intestine. *E. zurnii:* Throughout small intestine, cecum, colon, and rectum.

Identification: *E. bovis:* Oval with a mean size of 20 x 28 μ. Sporulation time is 48-72 hours at room temperature. *E. auburnensis:* Elongate oval, size about 37 x 23 μ. Sporulation time 48-72 hours at room temperature. *E. zurnii:* Vary from subspherical to ellipsoidal, about 15 x 18 μ in size, sporulation time about 72 hours at room temperature.

Distribution and importance: Widespread throughout North America and of major economic importance to the cattle industry. Severe losses in dairy calves and feeder cattle may be due to these protozoans.

Life cycle: In general, similar to life cycle of *E. tenella.*

Transmission: Ingestion of sporulated oocyst with food or water.

Signs and pathogenicity: *E. zurnii* and *E. bovis* are the coccidia usually associated with clinical coccidiosis in cattle. *E. auburnensis* is common in North American cattle, but it is less pathogenic than the other two species. In general, infections are seen in young stock a few weeks to 6 months old. Under certain conditions it may be seen in yearlings and adults if massive numbers of oocysts are ingested.

Serious losses may occur if dairy calves are overcrowded and kept in unsanitary conditions. Outbreaks of the disease may occur in feedlot and yarded cattle. Such an outbreak in winter is often referred to as winter coccidiosis. Presumably the manure and bedding provide sufficient heat and moisture for oocyst sporulation even in freezing weather. Introduction of new shipments of calves to a lot where the infection has built up over several months may be followed by an explosive outbreak of fatal coccidiosis. In acute outbreaks of the disease hemorrhagic diarrhea is a common clinical sign; oocysts usually can be demonstrated in large numbers. However, in peracute cases, there may be few oocysts. The developing stages may damage the epithelium before oocysts are produced and shed.

Diagnosis: Based on clinical signs and the demonstration of large numbers of oocysts. At necropsy, scrapings of the intestinal mucosae should reveal many developing stages of coccidia.

Control: Good management, sanitation, and hygiene are helpful in preventing coccidiosis. Overstocking and crowding should be avoided, and fecal contamination of feeders and waterers should be prevented as far as is practical. Dairy calves should be isolated in individual pens that are cleaned daily. Slat-bottom pens are recommended to help maintain cleanliness. Portable pens for outdoor use can be moved weekly to clean ground. Sunlight is always helpful in the destruction of unsporulated oocysts.

Immunity seems to develop to some species of bovine coccidia but is variable among strains of coccidia within a species. The precise nature of resistance to reinfection is still not clearly understood. For treatment, the sulfonamides are of some value. Treatment of animals with advanced clinical signs may respond very little to any type of medication. Spontaneous recovery may occur in spite of medication. Amprolium is claimed to be quite effective when administered over a prolonged period in the feed.

Selected references:

Davis, L. R., and G. W. Bowman. 1952. Coccidiosis of cattle. *Proc. U. S. Livestock San. Assoc.* 58th Ann. meeting. Pp. 39-50.
———. 1957. The endogenous development of *Eimeria zurnii*, a pathogenic coccidium of cattle. *Am. J. Vet. Res.* 18:569-74.
Fitzgerald, P. R. 1972. The economics of bovine coccidiosis. *Feedstuffs* 44:28-29.

PARASITE: *Eimeria debliecki* (coccidia)

Disease: Coccidiosis (porcine).
Host: Domestic and wild pigs.
Habitat: Small intestine.
Identification: Several coccidia have been reported from the pig. The descriptions of these species are based only on oocysts in the feces. *E. debliecki* is probably the most common coccidium of the pig. The oocysts are ovoid and about 17 x 25 μ.

Distribution and importance: Widely distributed, its importance has not been fully evaluated.

Life cycle: Endogenous cycle takes place in the small intestine, usually in the jejunum and ileum. In general the life cycle follows the usual coccidial pattern; sporulation is claimed to take 96-216 hours, longer than for most coccidia.

Transmission: Ingestion of sporulated oocysts with contaminated food or water.

Signs and pathogenicity: The pathogenicity of this protozoan is questionable. *E. debliecki* does not seem to be associated with clinical signs of disease in mature hogs. Young pigs experimentally fed large numbers of oocysts were severely diarrheic, stunted, emaciated, and there was some mortality. The older pig appears to serve as the carrier.

Diagnosis: Based on clinical observations and the demonstration of oocysts in the feces or endogenous forms from the small intestine.

Control: Oocysts may remain viable in soil for 15 months. Use of runs and pastures must be carefully planned, and sanitation of pens is very important. Treatment of hog coccidiosis has received little attention. Sulfonamides appear to have prophylactic value and reduce oocyst production.

Selected references:

Alicata, J. E., and E. L. Willett. 1946. Observations on the prophylactic and curative value of sulfaguanidine in swine coccidiosis. *Am. J. Vet. Res.* 7:94-100.

Vetterling, J. M. 1965. Coccidia (Protozoa: Eimeriidae) of swine. *J. Parasitol.* 51: 897-912.

———. 1966. Endogenous cycle of the swine coccidium *Eimeria debliecki* Douwes, 1921. *J. Protozool.* 13:290-300.

PARASITE: *Eimeria magna*, *E. perforans* (coccidia)

Disease: Intestinal coccidiosis (lapine).

Host: Domestic and wild rabbit.

Habitat: From lower duodenum to lower ileum.

Identification: *E. magna:* Oocysts ellipsoidal and yellow to brown; mean size 35-24 μ. Sporulation time is 2-3 days. *E. perforans:* Oocysts ellipsoidal, colorless to pinkish; mean size 26 x 16 μ. Sporulation time is 48 hours.

Distribution and importance: Reported mostly from California. With good management it is not a disease of major importance.

Life cycle: Follows the general pattern of *E. tenella*.

Transmission: Ingestion of food and water contaminated with sporulated oocysts.

Signs and pathogenicity: *E. magna* is generally considered one of the more pathogenic of the intestinal coccidia of the rabbit; *E. perforans* is one of the less pathogenic species. Usual signs are inappetence, weight loss, diarrhea, and potbelly. Epithelial sloughing may occur.

Diagnosis: Demonstration of large numbers of oocysts in the feces.

Control: See *E. stiedai*; essentially based on good management practices. Regular and thorough cleaning of cages is of utmost significance.

Selected references:

Davies, S. F. M., L. P. Joyner, and S. B. Kendall. 1963. *Coccidiosis*. Edinburgh and London: Oliver and Boyd.

Horton-Smith, C. 1947. Treatment of hepatic coccidiosis in rabbits. *Vet. J.* 103:207-13.

McPherson, C. W., R. T. Haberman, R. R. Every, and R. Pierson. 1962. Eradication of intestinal coccidiosis from a large breeding colony of rabbits. *Proc. An. Care Panel* 12:133-40.

PARASITE: *Eimeria meleagridis*, *E. meleagrimitis*, *E. adenoeides* (coccidia)

Disease: Intestinal coccidiosis (turkey).

Host: Domestic and wild turkey.

Habitat: Small intestine and cecum (*E. meleagridis*); upper jejunum (*E. meleagrimitis*); cecum (*E. adenoeides*).

Identification: *E. meleagridis:* Oocysts ellipsoidal with mean size of 24 x 17 μ. Sporulation time is 24 hours, prepatent period is 96-120 hours. *E. meleagrimitis:* Oocyst subspherical, mean size about 19 x 16 μ and sporulation time 24-48 hours. *E. adenoeides:* Oocyst ovoid with a mean size of 26 x 17 μ. Sporulation time reported to be 20-98 hours.

Distribution and importance: Widely distributed throughout North America. Annual loss to turkey industry in the U.S. is about 1 million dollars.

Life cycle: Similar to general life cycle for coccidia (See *E. tenella*).

Transmission: Ingestion of sporulated oocyst with food and water.

Signs and pathogenicity: Severity of the disease depends on the number of oocysts ingested. Little pathogenicity is attributed to *E. meleagridis*, whereas *E. meleagrimitis* and *E. adenoeides* may be quite harmful. Generally the disease is most often seen in young birds. Infected birds stop eating, huddle together, and pass fluid droppings which may be brown or blood tinged.

In infections of *E. meleagrimitis* lesions appear about 4 days after infection. The jejunum becomes thickened and contains colorless fluid and mucus, small amounts of blood, and other cellular material. On the 5th or 6th day the duodenum becomes involved, the blood vessels are engorged, and a necrotic core may develop. The small intestine becomes congested and has petechial hemorrhages throughout. In *E. adenoeides* a severe enteritis with petechiae may occur about the 4th day postinfection. Feces may be fluid and blood-tinged, and contain mucous casts; occasionally caseous plugs are found in the ceca.

Diagnosis: At necropsy the location of lesions usually indicates the species of coccidia involved. Measurement of the oocyst and observation of the sporulation time are helpful in specific identification.

Control: See suggested control measures for *E. tenella*. Appropriate treatment agents are sulfonamides or amprolium.

Selected references:

Clarkson, M. J., and M. A. Gentles. 1958. Coccidiosis in turkeys. *Vet. Rec.* 70:211-14.

Hawkins, P. A. 1952. Coccidiosis in turkeys. *Mich. Agr. Expt. Sta. Bul.* 226:1-87.

Joyner, L. P. 1973. Coccidiosis in turkeys and its control. *Folia Vet. Latina.* 3:110-23.

PARASITE: *Eimeria necatrix, E. acervulina, E. maxima, E. mitis, E. praecox, E. hagani, E. mivati, E. brunetti* (coccidia)

Disease: Avian coccidiosis, intestinal coccidiosis.

Host: Chicken.

Habitat: *E. necatrix* is usually located in the anterior or midportion of the gut. *E. brunetti* is found in the lower small intestine, rectum, cecum, or cloaca. *E. acervulina, E. mivati, E. hagani, E. mitis,* and *E. praecox* are all found in the upper half of the small intestine.

Identification: The species of *Eimeria* in the small intestine differ only slightly in their size and general morphology. For practical reasons they can be arbitrarily differentiated according to the location of the lesions in the digestive tract. Approximate sizes of oocysts in microns are:

E. necatrix	20 x 17	*E. praecox*	21 x 17
E. acervulina	17 x 14	*E. hagani*	19 x 18
E. maxima	30 x 21	*E. mivati*	16 x 13
E. mitis	16 x 16	*E. brunetti*	24 x 20

Distribution and importance: Generally encountered throughout North America. Each species varies in its ability to produce disease.

Life cycle: In general the life cycle is similar to that of *E. tenella*.

Transmission: Ingestion of contaminated food or water.

Signs and pathogenicity: The intestinal forms of coccidia are quite variable in their ability to produce disease. Complex interrelationships between host and parasite seem to exist. These relationships are influenced by factors such as environment, nutrition, and management. Usual signs of the disease are decreased feed intake, increased water consumption, weight loss, and a fall in egg production if laying birds are involved. A catarrhal enteritis is usual as is a thickened intestinal wall. The intestinal lumen may be filled with clotted or unclotted blood; petechial hemorrhages are present. Intestinal epithelium may slough and be replaced by connective tissue that interferes with intestinal absorption. Some species seem to provoke a catarrhal and necrotic enteritis and coagulation necrosis. Circumcumscribed white spots may be seen through the mucosa; on microscopic examination, these are seen to contain developing coccidial forms.

Diagnosis: At necropsy, a diagnosis should be based on demonstration of coccidial forms from characteristic lesions in specific locations in the intestine. Coccidial forms are not always easy to demonstrate.

Control: Similar to the procedures suggested for *E. tenella*. Preventive medication consists of continuous use of anticoccidials in feed and water. These include the sulfonamides, nitrofurazones, nicarbazin, pyrimidine derivatives, and others. Vaccination has been practiced with concurrent use of sulfonamides. Vaccination, though recommended, has not been widely adopted as a preventive procedure.

Selected references:

Davies, S. F. M. 1956. Intestinal coccidiosis in chickens caused by *Eimeria necatrix*. *Vet. Rec.* 68:853-57.

Joyner, L. P., and P. L. Long. 1974. The specific characters of the *Eimeria* with special reference to the coccidia of the fowl. *Avian Pathology*. 3:145-57.

Levine, N. D. 1973. *Protozoan parasites of domestic animals and of man*. 2nd ed. Minneapolis: Burgess. Pp. 197-207 and 236-43.

Proc. of Symposium on Coccidia and Related Organisms. 1973. Univ. of Guelph, Ontario, Canada. Pp. 1-134.

Reid, W. M. 1964. A diagnostic chart for nine species of fowl coccidia. *Georgia Agr. Expt. Sta. Tech. Bul.* N.S. 39:5-18.

PARASITE: *Eimeria ninakohlyakimovae, E. ovina* (syn.: *arloingi*), *E. parva*. Of a dozen coccidian species reported for sheep and goats, these appear to be the more important.

Disease: Coccidiosis (ovine).

Host: Domestic and wild sheep and goats.

Habitat: *E. ninakohlyakimovae:* small intestine, ileum, and cecum. *E. ovina:* small intestine. *E. parvae:* small intestine, cecum, and colon.

Identification: *E. ninakohlyakimovae:* subspherical oocysts, about 22 x 19 μ;

sporulation time 24-96 hours; prepatent period 11-15 days. *E. ovina (arloingi):* ellipsoidal to oval oocysts, sides somewhat straight, about 30 x 20 μ; sporulation time 48-96 hours; prepatent period about 19 days. *E. parva:* oocysts variable but generally subspherical, about 17 x 14 μ; sporulation time 24-48 hours.

Distribution and importance: Widespread throughout the U.S. and of major importance to the feedlot lamb industry.

Life cycle: In general, similar to that of *E. tenella*. The disease is usually seen 2-3 weeks after a new shipment of lambs arrives in the feedlot.

Transmission: Ingestion of sporulated oocysts with food and water.

Signs and pathogenicity: Dependent upon the number of infective oocysts ingested and the pathogenicity of the coccidian species. *E. ninakohlyakimovae* is one of the more pathogenic coccidia of sheep; *E. ovina* is less pathogenic, whereas *E. parva* apparently is relatively harmless. Clinical signs are diarrhea, depression, inappetence, weakness, and weight loss. Mortality is seldom greater than 10%. There may be considerable weight loss and reduction in weight gains.

Diagnosis: Usually based on history, signs, gross lesions, and the demonstration of coccidial stages in intestinal smears taken at necropsy. Coccidial oocysts in feces indicate the presence of coccidia but not necessarily clinical coccidiosis.

Control: Management and good sanitation are the keys to prevention. Feedlots should be well drained and kept dry. Water troughs and feed racks should be raised to avoid contamination with feces as much as is practical. Severe freezing of the soil cannot be relied upon to kill unsporulated oocysts on pasture or in the feedlot. Sunlight and desiccation are valuable in the destruction of oocysts. Little information about the satisfactory treatment of ovine coccidiosis is available. No curative treatments are available. Sulfur, 0.15-1.5%, fed in chopped alfalfa and ground corn bound together by molasses and water is claimed to prevent coccidiosis in feeder lambs. Amprolium has shown promise in controlling clinical coccidiosis due to *E. ninakohlyakimovae.*

Selected references:

Landers, E. J. 1953. The effect of low temperatures upon the viability of unsporulated oocysts of ovine coccidia. *J. Parasitol.* 39:547-52.

Lotze, J. C. 1952. The pathogenicity of the coccidian parasite *E. arloingi*, in domestic sheep. *Cornell Vet.* 42:510-17.

———. 1953. Life history of the coccidian parasite, *E. arloingi* in domestic sheep. *Am. J. Vet. Res.* 14:86-95.

———. 1953. The pathogenicity of the coccidian parasite, *Eimeria ninakohlyakimovae*, Yakimov and Rastegaeva, 1930, in domestic sheep. *Proc. Am. Vet. Med. Assoc.* 141-46.

Pont, D. D. 1969. Coccidiosis of sheep. *Vet. Bul.* 39:609-18.
Salisbury, R. M., and L. K. Whitten. 1953. Coccidiosis of sheep—a review. *N. Z. Vet. J.* 1:69-72.

PARASITE: *Eimeria stiedai* (coccidian)

Disease: Hepatic coccidiosis (lapine).

Host: Domestic and wild rabbit.

Habitat: Epithelial cells of the bile ducts.

Identification: Oocysts are oval, slightly pink, and mean size is 37 x 21 μ. The micropyle is distinct. Sporulation time is about 72 hours.

Distribution and importance: Widely distributed throughout the U.S. It is important to commercial rabbit producers and pet owners.

Life cycle: On ingestion with food and water, sporulated oocysts excyst, and the liberated sporozoites penetrate the intestinal mucosa, enter the hepatic portal circulation, and are carried to the liver. Here they parasitize the epithelial cells of the bile ducts and grow to schizonts that produce merozoites. The latter multiply asexually for an indefinite number of generations ultimately producing gametocytes. Oocysts are produced and pass into the intestine with the bile and onto the ground in droppings. The prepatent period is 6-9 days.

Transmission: Ingestion of sporulated oocysts with contaminated food and water.

Signs and pathogenicity: In light infections there may be no clinical signs. In severe cases inappetence and emaciation may occur. The disease is usually spectacular in young rabbits; death may occur in 2-3 weeks. The disease may also be chronic. Clinical signs are usually associated with liver dysfunction. The liver may become greatly enlarged with circular, creamy nodules and elongate cordlike structures throughout the parenchyma. Biliary hyperplasia is extensive. Scrapings from the bile duct lesions usually contain masses of coccidial forms.

Diagnosis: Characteristic hepatic lesions on necropsy. Demonstration of coccidial forms from the cheesy content of early liver lesions or demonstration of oocysts on fecal examination.

Control: Basically accomplished by good management. Feeders and waterers should be designed and located to remain uncontaminated by feces. Equipment must be kept scrupulously clean. Cage flooring should be hardware cloth to allow feces to fall through. As a prophylactic measure, sulfaquinoxaline may be given continuously in a concentration of 0.025% for 30 days. For therapeutic control, a concentration of 0.10% sulfaquinoxaline in feed for 2 weeks is effective. Alternatively, 0.05% sulfaquinoxaline in the feed and 0.04% in the drinking water given continuously for 2 weeks will effect control.

Selected references:

Horton-Smith, C. 1947. Treatment of hepatic coccidiosis in rabbits. *Vet. J.* 103:207-13.

Lund, E. E. 1949. Considerations on the practical control of intestinal coccidiosis of domestic rabbits. *Ann. N. Y. Acad. Sci.* 52:611-20.

McPherson, C. W., R. T. Haberman, R. R. Every, and R. Pierson. 1962. Eradication of intestinal coccidiosis from a large breeding colony of rabbits. *Proc. An. Care Panel* 12:133-40.

PARASITE: *Eimeria tenella* (coccidia)

Disease: Cecal coccidiosis (chicken).

Host: Chicken.

Habitat: Cecum.

Identification: Oocysts are broadly oval with a mean size of 23 x 19 μ. Sporulation time is 24-48 hours.

Distribution and importance: Widely distributed throughout the U.S. It is of major economic importance to the poultry industry because it is highly pathogenic and responsible for heavy financial loss.

Life cycle: Oocysts are passed in the feces; sporulation occurs on the ground with sporoblast formation. Four sporoblasts develop into sporocysts each producing 2 sporozoites. The oocyst is then infective. When the sporulated oocyst is ingested, the sporozoites are released, and they enter the cecal epithelium and become first-generation schizonts. Asexual reproduction follows, producing merozoites. Repeated schizogony may occur; then the sexual stage of the life cycle is initiated. The prepatent period is 6 days.

Transmission: Ingestion of sporulated oocysts with food or water.

Signs and pathogenicity: Disease most frequently seen in younger birds of 4-6 weeks old. Depending on size of infective dose, cecal coccodiosis may be an inapparent infection, but usually it is a highly fatal disease. It is frequently an acute disease with diarrhea and massive cecal hemorrhage. Blood is seen in the droppings 4 days after the initial infection. The birds become listless, eat little, and are notably thirsty. Massive cecal hemorrhage is seen on the 5th and 6th days after infection. Maximum oocyst production occurs about the 7th day if the bird survives. If the bird remains alive until the 8th or 9th day after infection, it usually recovers. Lesions commonly seen are extensive epithelial sloughing and a cecum filled with partially clotted blood that ultimately consolidates to form cecal cores. The wall of the cecum becomes markedly thickened and enlarged, and a severe anemia may occur because of blood loss.

Diagnosis: By demonstration of oocysts from feces or mucosal scrapings at necropsy. Findings must be interpreted with care. The presence of oocysts does not always indicate that the clinical signs are caused by the coccidia; conversely, clinical signs may be present, but it may be difficult to demonstrate oocysts. In cecal coccidiosis, the clinical signs are usually spectacular.

Control: Coccidial oocysts are generally resistant to environmental extremes. They may remain viable for a year or more under suitable conditions of moisture and temperature. Eventually they are killed by subfreezing temperatures. Commonly used antiseptics and disinfectants have little effect on the oocyst. Under most farm conditions it is almost impossible to prevent birds from acquiring a few oocysts. Prevention of clinical coccidiosis consists of preventing a heavy enough infection to produce disease and, at the same time, allowing the production of an asymptomatic infection to develop immunity. This may be accomplished by good management and sanitation supplemented by coccidiostatic medication in feed or water.

Young birds should be raised apart from older birds. If deep litter is used, it should be forked over, mixed well, and kept dry. Feeders and waterers should be thoroughly cleaned weekly and kept on wire platforms to prevent fecal contamination. The use of a coccidiosis vaccine is claimed to be a successful method of immunizing chickens. It is a suspension of sporulated oocysts of many species and is given in the feed at 3-5 days of age. An anticoccidial is fed at the same time and continued until 5 weeks after the initial vaccination. Though vaccination works well under certain conditions, failures have been reported, and the program has never been widely adopted for routine use. Many anticoccidials are effective in preventing infections, but they have little value in treatment. For treatment the most commonly used drugs are the sulfonamides and amprolium. These drugs may be given in feed or water. Inevitably, as a result of using anticoccidials in feed over a long period, drug-resistant strains develop. Periodically the anticoccidial should be changed. Preventive measures without complete reliance on drugs seems to be the most prudent program to follow.

Selected references:

Joyner, L. P. 1964. Coccidiosis in the domestic fowl. *Vet. Bul.* 34:311-15.

Reid, W. M. 1973. Anticoccidials: differences in day of peak activity against *E. tenella*. Proc. Symposium on Coccidia and Related Organisms. Univ. of Guelph, Ontario, Canada. Pp. 119-34.

PARASITE: *Eimeria truncata* (coccidia)

Disease: Renal coccidiosis.
Host: Domestic and wild goose, duck.

Habitat: Epithelial cells of kidney tubules.

Identification: Oocysts ovoid, about 19 x 14 μ, with a narrow, small end. Sporulation time is 24-120 hours.

Distribution and importance: Appears to be widely distributed. As far as is known, it is not of great economic importance.

Life cycle: Schizonts seen in epithelial cells of the kidney tubules, prepatent period 5-6 days. Life cycle is not known in detail.

Transmission: Ingestion of sporulated oocysts with contaminated food and water. Wild geese may be responsible for introduction of an infection.

Signs and pathogenicity: A pathogen for goslings. Disease may be acute with 100% mortality. Affected birds are weak and emaciated. The kidneys have white nodules or streaks on the surface and throughout the parenchyma. Tubules may be packed with urates, and oocysts and coccidial forms in various stages of development are seen.

Diagnosis: Demonstration of oocyst and other forms from infected kidney tissues.

Control: No specific recommendations other than rigid sanitation and hygiene. No treatment is available.

Selected references:

Critcher, S. 1950. Renal coccidiosis in Pea Island Canada geese. *Wildlife N. Carolina.* 14:14-15.

Hanson, H. C., N. D. Levine, and V. Ivens. 1957. Coccidia of North American wild geese and swans. *Can J. Zool.* 35:715-33.

Stubbs, E. L. 1957. Case report—renal coccidiosis in geese. *Avian Dis.* 1:349.

PARASITE: *Entamoeba coli* (nonpathogenic amoeba)

Disease: Entamoebiasis.

Host: Man, occasionally dog and other animals.

Habitat: Large intestine.

Identification: Trophozoites are 15-50 μ and move very sluggishly. The cyst form is 15-30 μ in diameter and has 1-8 distinct nuclei; 8 nuclei are characteristic of the mature cyst.

Distribution and importance: Is important because it must be differentiated from *E. histolytica*. Incidence in man is about 30% in the U.S.; incidence in other animals is not known.

Life cycle: The life cycle parallels that of *E. histolytica* and involves precystic, cyst, metacyst, and trophozoite forms.

Transmission: By ingestion of the mature cysts.

Signs and pathogenicity: No signs observed. This lumen parasite is nonpathogenic.

Diagnosis: Identification of trophozoites in the fresh, loose stool or the mature cyst with more than 4 nuclei. The cyst must be carefully differentiated from that of *E. histolytica*.

Control: Not indicated. The presence of *E. coli* suggests that feces have been introduced into the mouth. Sanitation and hygiene should be stressed.

Selected references:

Dobell, C. 1938. Researches on the intestinal protozoa of monkeys and man. IX. The life history of *E. coli* with special reference to metacystic development. *Parasitology* 30:195-238.

PARASITE: *Entamoeba histolytica* (amoeba)

Disease: Entamoebiasis (canine).

Host: *E. histolytica:* man, primates, dog, cat, pig and rat. *E. equi, E. gedoelsti:* horse. *E. bovis:* cattle. *E: suis:* pig. *E. cuniculi:* rabbit. The species in the horse and cow are generally considered nonpathogenic for these hosts.

Habitat: Large intestine, sometimes liver.

Identification: The active trophozoite is 10-60 μ depending on the variety. The cyst is 10-20 μ in diameter with a wall about 0.5 μ thick. Characteristically not more than 4 nuclei are in the mature cyst. Trophozoites (*E. histolytica*) may contain ingested erythrocytes.

Distribution and importance: Reported incidence in dogs from Louisiana is 7-10% and from Tennessee is 8.4%. In the U.S. incidence in man is about 2.0%.

Life cycle: Trophozoites multiply in the large intestine by binary fission. Before expulsion from the host, the amoebae become round, lay down a cyst wall, and encyst. Within the cyst the nucleus divides to form, characteristically, 4 nuclei. Following ingestion, 4 nucleate amoebae emerge; the nuclei and cytoplasm divide, resulting in 8 small amoebulae that develop into trophozoites.

Transmission: Through ingestion of contaminated food or water.

Signs and pathogenicity: In the dog a chronic disease with indefinite signs is usually associated with infections of *E. histolytica*. Proteolytic enzymes produced by trophozoites may cause local dissolution of tissues and lysis of epithelium. Diarrhea and dysentery may occur, and flask shaped areas on the walls of the cecum and colon may become ulcerated. The kitten appears to be especially susceptible to this protozoan and has an acute amoebic dysentery with ulcerations of the bowel wall. In both the cat and dog, encystment generally does not occur. Manifestations of the disease in the dog vary from a mild diarrhea with spontaneous recovery to a fulminating dysentery and death.

Diagnosis: Usually accomplished by the examination of fresh, *warm* feces for trophozoites or—if the feces are old, preserved, or held under refrigeration —for cysts. The fresh trophozoite may contain ingested red blood cells, helpful in differentiating *E. histolytica* from other amoebae. The mature cyst of *E. histolytica* is characterized by 4 nuclei. However in the dog and cat, the cyst form is rarely seen; a diagnosis rests on the demonstration of the trophozoite form. Experimentally it has been shown that feeding raw liver or cod liver oil to dogs infected with *E. histolytica* induces encystment of the trophozoites.

Control: It is improbable that humans can be infected with *E. histolytica* from other animals, for they pass only the trophozoite stage. However, man releases cysts that are resistant and infective for other species. Strict sanitation and hygiene are important. Avoid fecal contamination of food and water supplies. The common amoebicides used in man, such as diodoquin, carbarsone, emetine hydrochloride, and metronidazole, may be tried on animals.

Selected references:

Hoare, C. A. 1959. Amoebic infections in animals. *Vet. Rev. Annotations* 5:91-102.

Jordan, H. E. 1967. Amebiasis (*Entamoeba histolytica*) in the dog. *Vet. Med. Small Anim. Clin.* 62:61-64.

Thorson, R. E., H. E. Siebold, and W. S. Bailey. 1956. Systemic amebiasis with distemper in a dog. *J. Am. Vet. Med. Assoc.* 129:335-37.

Wittnich, C. 1976. *Entamoeba histolytica* infection in a German shepherd dog. *Can. Vet. Jour.* 17:259-62.

PARASITE: *Giardia canis*, *G. cati* (flagellate)

Disease: Giardiasis.

Host: Dog, cat (*G. cati*).

Habitat: Duodenum, jejunum.

Identification: Vegetative form is pyriform to ellipsoidal and bilaterally symmetrical. A large sucking disc is present on the ventral surface. Two anterior nuclei are readily seen; 8 flagella are present. Trophozoite may be 17 μ long and about 10 μ wide. Cyst is oval, about 10 by 8 μ, and with 2-4 nuclei.

Distribution and importance: Probably widespread throughout the U.S. Importance as a disease agent is still undetermined.

Life cycle: Reproduction is by binary fission.

Transmission: By ingestion of food or water contaminated with cysts. The cyst may remain viable for about 2 weeks in moist surroundings.

Signs and pathogenicity: The pathogenicity of this parasite for dogs is still controversial. Diarrhea has been described for a number of young, infected dogs, but the organism has not been demonstrated as responsible for this condition.

Diagnosis: Identification of the cyst from the feces.

Control: Strict sanitation is essential. Quinacrine, 50-100 mg., t.i.d. for 2-3 days has been shown to be effective. Metronidazole (Flagyl) is also recommended. It has been suggested that an animal on a high carbohydrate diet is more susceptible to *G. canis* than one on a high protein diet.

Selected references:

Catcott, E. J. 1946. The incidence of intestinal protozoa in the dog. *J. Am. Vet. Med. Assoc.* 108:34-36.

Choquette, L. P. E., and L. de G. Gelinas. 1950. The incidence of intestinal nematodes and protozoa in dogs in the Montreal district. *Can. J. Comp. Med. Vet. Sci.* 14:33-38.

Craige, J. E. 1949. Intestinal disturbance in dogs; differential diagnosis and therapy. *J. Am. Vet. Med. Assoc.* 114:425-28.

PARASITE: *Haemoproteus columbae* (haemosporidian)

Disease: Haemoproteiasis.

Host: Pigeons, doves, and many other columboid wild birds.

Habitat: Gametocytes occur in erythrocytes. Schizogony takes place in endothelial cells of the blood vessels.

Identification: Mature gametocytes are elongate or sausage-shaped, frequently partially encircling the nucleus of the host cell.

Distribution and importance: Widespread throughout North America; not generally considered of major economic importance.

Life cycle: Bird infected when bit by the arthropod vector. Sporozoites enter the blood vessels of lung, liver, and spleen. Schizonts form cytomeres. Cytomeres ultimately produce large numbers of merozoites which enter the bloodstream. Following schizogony, the merozoites enter the red blood cells and ultimately become micro- or macrogametes.

Transmission: By bite of the infected hippoboscid fly *Pseudolynchia* sp.

Signs and pathogenicity: Infected birds usually show no signs of disease.

Diagnosis: Demonstration of the organisms in stained blood smears. Parasites observed must be differentiated from forms of *Plasmodium*.

Control: Not generally undertaken; treatment does not seem necessary. Screening against hippoboscid flies may be attempted.

Selected references:

Herman, C. M. 1954. *Haemoproteus* infections in waterfowl. *Proc. Helminthol. Soc. Wash.* 21:37-42.

PARASITE: *Hexamita meleagridis* (flagellate)

Disease: Hexamitiasis (infectious catarrhal enteritis).

Host: Turkey, chicken, duck, and many wild birds; Usually in younger birds.

Habitat: Duodenum, small intestine.

Identification: Body is pyriform with 6 anterior and 2 posterior flagellae. Mean size is 9 x 3 μ. Movement is rapid and jerky without spiraling.

Distribution and importance: Widely distributed through North America. The importance of this disease has not been evaluated.

Life cycle: Multiplication by longitudinal fission.

Transmission: By ingesting freshly contaminated food or water.

Signs and pathogenicity: Adult birds are frequently asymptomatic carriers; usually a disease of turkey poults less than 10 weeks old. Poults appear nervous and have a stilted gait and ruffled feathers. Birds lose weight rapidly, become weak and listless, and die. Incubation period is 4-7 days. Necropsy shows a severe catarrhal inflammation of the intestine. Intestinal contents are thin and watery; a white foamy diarrhea is often present.

Diagnosis: Demonstration of the organism in *fresh* scrapings from the mucosa of the small intestine, particularly the duodenum and jejunum. This protozoan is very delicate and disintegrates rapidly after death of its host.

Control: Prevention consists of good management and strict sanitation. Poults should be separated from adults; feeders and waterers should be on wire platforms to prevent contamination. No treatment has been consistently successful. Replacement of drinking water for several days with a mixture of 3% dried whey in 1:2000 aqueous copper sulfate solution has been claimed to be efficacious. Enheptin is also said to be useful therapeutically, and Di-n-butyl tin dilaurate has shown promise as a protozoacide.

Selected references:

Levine, N. D., P. D. Beamer, and C. E. McNeil. 1952. *Hexamita* from the golden pheasant. *J. Parasitol.* 38:90.

PARASITE: *Histomonas meleagridis*

Disease: Histomoniasis, blackhead, infectious enterohepatitis.

Host: Turkey, chicken, guinea fowl, peahen, pheasant, and other wild birds.

Habitat: Lumen of cecum and parenchyma of liver and cecum.

Identification: This protozoan is pleomorphic. Tissue forms are amoeboid; those found in the lumen or free in contents of the cecum may be elonate with a single flagellum. The amoeboid forms are 8-15 μ in diameter; those free in the lumen may be from 5-30 μ in diameter. Organism rotates counterclockwise in a jerky, rhythmic motion.

Distribution and importance: Widely distributed throughout North America and of major import in turkey-raising areas.

Life cycle: Reproduction is by binary fission. There is no cyst. Trophozoites are delicate and do not survive more than a few hours in feces. *H. mele-ogridis* in the lumen of the cecum of the host is ingested by the cecal worm *Heterakis gallinarum.* It penetrates the intestinal wall of the worm, reaches the ovary, and enters the worm egg. The cecal worm egg carrying the histomonad is then ingested by another bird, whereupon the egg hatches releasing a worm larva. This larva irritates the cecal mucosa and the protozoan then becomes established.

Transmission: Usually by ingestion of infected egg of *H. gallinarum.* Infection may also occur through ingestion of large numbers of infective trophozoites in very fresh droppings. Infected cecal worm eggs may remain viable for 1-2 years in soil. Trophozoites do not survive more than a few hours in feces. Earthworms may also serve as mechanical carriers for infected cecal worm eggs.

Signs and pathogenicity: Turkeys of any age may be affected. The disease is most often seen in birds 3-12 weeks old; losses may be 50% or more. Chickens are much less susceptible than turkeys, and ordinarily chickens are asymptomatic. The first signs of disease are weakness and drowsiness; birds stand with heads lowered, droopy wings, and closed eyes. They do not eat and lose weight, and the droppings may be sulfur-colored. The incubation period is 2-3 weeks. The concave liver lesions are pathognomic and are saucer-shaped, depressed, yellow-green areas of necrosis and degeneration. They are 1-2 cm. in diameter. Cecal lesions are first seen as pinpoint ulcers that enlarge and appear as yellow patches on the serosal surface. The lumen of the cecum may contain a hard caseous core to which the cecal epithelium adheres.

Diagnosis: Usually made when characteristic liver lesions are seen on necropsy of a bird that has died recently.

Control: The disease can be prevented by good management. The cardinal rule is to keep chickens completely separate from turkeys. Turkeys should be placed in clean runs that have not been used for at least 10 months and preferably for 2 years. Turkeys must not be placed on ground that has been fertilized with chicken or turkey manure. Continuous feeding of a ration containing enheptin or hepzidé has proved satisfactory in prevention of the disease. This chemical may also be used therapeutically. Range rotation should be practiced routinely. Feeders and waterers should be kept off the ground and on wire platforms.

Selected references:

Gibbs, B. J. 1962. The occurrence of the protozoan parasite *Histomonas meleagridis* in the adults and eggs of the cecal worm *Heterakis gallinae. J. Protozool.* 9:288-93.

Lund, E. E. 1969. Histomoniasis. *Adv. Vet. Sci.* 13:355-90.

Reid, W. M. 1967. Etiology and dissemination of the blackhead disease syndrome in turkeys and chickens. *Exp. Parasitol.* 21:249-75.

Wehr, E. E., M. M. Farr, and D. K. McLaughlin. 1958. Chemotherapy of blackhead in poultry. *J. Am. Vet. Med. Assoc.* 132:439-45.

PARASITE: *Isospora bigemina, I. felis, I. canis, I. rivolta* (coccidia)

Disease: Intestinal coccidiosis (canine).

Host: Dog and cat (*I. bigemina*), cat (*I. felis*), dog (*I. canis*), dog and cat (*I. rivolta*).

Habitat: Small intestine, occasionally colon.

Identification: Developed oocyst contains 2 sporocysts each containing 4 sporozoites. Schizogony and gametogony take place within the host cells, and sporogony usually occurs outside the host's body. Mean sizes of oocysts in microns are as follows: *I. bigemina* — 13 x 10, *I. felis* — 42 x 31, *I. canis* — 38 x 20, *I. rivolta* — 23 x 19.

Distribution and importance: Widespread throughout North America. Death has been attributed to coccidia in pups and kittens; however, oocysts are often observed in these hosts without any evidence of clinical disease.

Life cycle: Developing stages are found throughout the small intestine. In acute infections the schizonts, gametocytes, and oocysts are found in epithelial cells. The prepatent period is 6-7 days. The oocyst is passed with the feces. In *Isospora* the sporulated oocyst develops 2 sporocysts, each of which contains 4 comma-shaped sporozoites. If ingested by a suitable host, the sporulated oocyst excysts and releases the sporozoites, which ultimately enter the intestinal epithelium and develop by undergoing schizogony and gametogony.

Transmission: Ingestion of sporulated (infective) oocyst, e.g., with food or water or from the hair coat or foot pads.

Signs and pathogenicity: Of the 4 species, *I. bigemina* seems to be the major pathogen for dogs and cats. In severe cases a catarrhal enteritis may become hemorrhagic, and feces may be blood-streaked. Emaciation and weakness are evident, and ultimately the victim may succumb. If the animal survives the acute stage, a gelatinous catarrhal enteritis may occur, and there may be signs of recovery in about 10 days. The other species are more benign and are often associated with a mild catarrhal enteritis.

Diagnosis: Based on clinical signs and the presence of many oocysts in the feces. Demonstration of developmental stages from mucosal scrapings at necropsy is a useful diagnostic procedure.

Control: The most important preventive procedures are cleanliness and good sanitation. Feces should be collected and removed at intervals shorter than that required for sporulation of the oocyst. Feeders and waterers should be kept scrupulously clean. No treatment is successful if signs of the disease have appeared. The anticoccidials available are preventive agents. Because the disease is self-limiting, many chemicals administered about the time of natural recovery have been credited with curative properties. Supportive treatment with antibiotics may help control secondary infection and indirectly help speed recovery.

Selected references:

Hitchcock, D. J. 1955. The life cycle of *Isospora felis* in the kitten. *J. Parasitol.* 41: 383-97.

Lee, C. D. 1934. The pathology of coccidiosis in the dog. *J. Am. Vet. Med. Assoc.* 85:760-81.

Shah, H. L. 1970. *Isospora* species of the cat and attempted transmission of *I. felis* Wenyon, 1923, from the cat to the dog. *J. Protozool.* 17:603-09.

———. 1971. The life cycle of *Isospora felis*, Wenyon, 1923, a coccidium of the cat. *J. Protozool.* 18:3-17.

PARASITE: *Leishmania donovani, L. tropica*

Disease: Leishmaniasis, kala azar, dumdum fever.

Host: Man, dog, cat, horse, and sheep.

Habitat: Found in reticulo-endothelial cells of capillaries, spleen, and other organs but may be seen in monocytes, polymorphonuclear leukocytes, and macrophages. *L. donovani* affects visceral areas, and *L. tropica* is found cutaneously.

Identification: Small intracellular, nonflagellated bodies are circular or oval, about 2 μ wide by 4 μ long. Occurs as a leptomonad in the insect host.

Distribution and importance: Not enzootic in North America. Four cases of canine leishmaniasis have been reported in the U.S. These were all in imported dogs. Canine leishmaniasis is prevalent in South America.

Life cycle: The leishmania organisms multiply by binary fission in reticulo-endothelial cells and macrophages. The dog may serve as a reservoir for the infective forms of this parasite, especially the Chinese, Mediterranean, and South American forms.

Transmission: Usually when bitten by an infected sand fly (*Phlebotomus* sp.) though other means of transmission are probable.

Signs and pathogenicity: The disease is chronic and is characterized by emaciation and general debility usually ending in death within a few years. Mortality is 70-90% in untreated animals. With treatment a 90% recovery may be anticipated. Animals frequently show a general anemia, enlarged liver, congested spleen, edema of the skin, and remittent fever.

Diagnosis: Usually by demonstrating organisms in smears on biopsy or at necropsy from the spleen, liver pulp, lymph nodes, or bone marrow.

Control: Protection against *Phlebotomus* sp. using screens and insecticides; destruction of stray and uncared-for dogs which may serve as reservoir hosts.

Selected references:

Adler, S. 1964. *Leishmania. Adv. Parasitol.* 2:35-69.

McConnell, E. E., E. F. Chaffee, I. G. Cashell, and F. M. Garner. 1970. Visceral leishmaniasis with ocular involvement in a dog. *J. Am. Vet. Med. Assoc.* 156:197-203.

Tryphonas, L., Z. Zawidzka, M. A. Bernard, and E. A. Janzen. 1977. Visceral leishmaniasis in a dog: clinical hematological and pathological observations. *Can. J. Comp. Med.* 41:1-12.

PARASITE: *Leucocytozoon simondi, L. smithi*

Disease: Leucocytozoonosis.

Host: Domestic and wild duck, geese (*L. simondi*); domestic and wild turkey (*L. smithi*).

Habitat: It is still uncertain which cells are parasitized especially in the case of *L. simondi*. Often the host cell is quite distorted by the parasite and cannot be readily identified. Mature gametocytes have been observed in monocytes, lymphocytes, and even erythrocytes. Schizogony occurs in the liver parenchyma and other organs.

Identification: In *L. simondi* the mature gametocytes are elongate and may be 22 μ long. The host cell is spindle- or cigar-shaped and as long as 50 μ. *L. smithi* is similar in size and morphology with the gametocyte about 22 μ long, the host cell is about 45 μ long.

Distribution and importance: Common throughout North America and important to commercial turkey and duck producers and to those who raise ducks on a farm pond or as a hobby.

Life cycle: Birds become infected when bitten by a blackfly vector. Sporozoites enter the bloodstream and invade various tissue cells where they develop to schizonts. In the duck, hepatic schizonts may be seen in the liver cells, or megaloschizonts may be found in the brain, lung, liver, heart, and other organs. The megaloschizonts eventually produce many thousands of merozoites which enter the bloodstream.

Transmission: By bite of an infected blackfly (*Simulium* spp.); many species are widely distributed throughout North America.

Signs and pathogenicity: *L. simondi* causes highly pathogenic disease in ducklings and goslings. Ducklings may appear well in the evening, be severely ill the following morning, and be dead by afternoon. Birds stop eating, become listless, show severe dyspnea, and die. Recovered birds remain carriers. Turkey poults infected with *L. smithi* lose their appetites, become droopy, and sit around. They may become incoordinated, keel over, and die. As with *L. simondi*, recovered birds remain carriers.

Diagnosis: By examination of blood smears and demonstration of the large spindle-shaped structures containing gametocytes.

Control: Blackfly control may be attempted but is difficult. Fine-mesh screening of poultry runs is expensive, and maintaining it is a problem. Turkeys and ducks should not be raised near fast-flowing water—the breeding grounds of the blackfly! Clopidol is claimed to be an effective treatment.

Selected references:

Bierer, B. W. 1950. Leucocytozoon infection in turkeys. *Vet. Med.* 45:87-88.

Fallis, A. M., D. M. Davies, and M. A. Vickers. 1951. Life history of *Leucocytozoon simondi* Mathis and Leger in natural and experimental infections and blood changes produced in the avian host. *Can. J. Zool.* 29:305-28.

Wehr, E. E. 1962. Studies on leucocytozoonosis of turkeys, with notes on schizogony, transmission and control of *Leucocytozoon smithi. Avian Dis.* 6:195-210.

PARASITE: *Pentatrichomonas* sp. (intestinal flagellate)

Disease: Pentatrichomoniasis (canine).

Host: Dog, usually puppies.

Habitat: Cecum, colon.

Identification: Size 8-12 μ long; usually has 5 anterior flagella though forms have been observed with 3 or 4.

Distribution and importance: Little known of its distribution or importance.

Life cycle: Multiplication is by simple fission.

Transmission: Trophozoites apparently can live outside the body long enough to be transferred to a new host.

Signs and pathogenicity: Some believe that *Pentatrichomonas* sp. is responsible for a persistent mucoid diarrhea sometimes associated with this protozoan in puppies. Clinical signs include diarrhea, anorexia, retarded growth, and rough hair coat in puppies 6-8 weeks old. Infections in mature dogs are considered asymptomatic.

Diagnosis: Preliminary diagnosis may be made by examination of a direct saline smear prepared from fresh feces or a rectal swab. Fresh feces may also be cultured. For detailed morphological study, the organisms should be fixed and stained.

Control: Treatment with metronidazole (Flagyl) has proved effective. Strict sanitation should be practiced at all times.

Selected references:

Buckner, R. G., and S. A. Ewing. 1971. Trichomoniasis. In *Current Veterinary Therapy*, IV, Small Animal Practice, ed. R. W. Kirk, pp. 582-83. Philadelphia: Saunders.

PARASITE: *Sarcocystis* spp. (sarcocyst)

Disease: Sarcosporidiosis (sarcocystosis).

Host: Not very host-specific; reported from many species of mammals and birds such as sheep, cattle, horse, pig, wild duck, and man.

Habitat: Striated and heart muscle, occasionally brain tissues.

Identification: At present the taxonomic status of *Sarcocystis* is uncertain. More than 50 species of this protozoan have been named, but their validity is questionable. Species are differentiated on the basis of host, cyst wall structure, and size of zoites. In general *Sarcocystis* apparently is not very host-specific. The cysts formerly known as Miescher's tubes are readily visible to the unaided eye and vary in size from a few mm. to 1 cm. or more in length. From the cyst wall, septa originate that divide the cyst into a number of compartments. When mature the cyst may be filled with banana-shaped spores (bradyzoites), about 10 x 4 μ. These were formerly known as Rainey's corpuscles, spores, or sporozoites.

Distribution and importance: Widespread throughout North America. In older meat-producing animals carcass condemnations may result in substantial economic loss.

Life cycle: At present the details of the life cycle are uncertain. The host becomes infected by ingesting trophozoites within cysts in the muscle or in the feces of animals. These forms are thought to pass through the intestinal wall, enter the bloodstream, and then invade the muscle cell. They are commonly found in the esophagus, tongue, masseter, diaphragm, and heart. In wild ducks they are usually seen in the breast muscle. According to Dubey, the carnivore is the definitive host, and the herbivore is an intermediate host. The definitive host becomes infected by ingesting the encysted stage of the parasite in the musculature of the intermediate host. The intermediate host acquires its infection by ingesting sporocysts or oocysts that are shed in the feces of infected definitive hosts. Sporozoites are released from the sporocysts in the intestine of the intermediate hosts and invade many tissues.

Transmission: Ingestion of infective muscle cysts or free trophozoites in the feces.

Signs and pathogenicity: This organism is not generally considered an important pathogen. Such things as lameness, emaciation, muscular stiffness, paralysis, and even death have been attributed to infections of *Sarcocystis*.

Cellular reaction to the cysts is usually minimal although focal myocarditis and myositis have been observed upon breakdown of the cysts. Cysts contain a potent endotoxin that is highly toxic when injected into rabbits, mice, and sparrows.

Diagnosis: Cysts are easily seen with the unaided eye. Examination of a histological section of the cyst will help in identification. Complement-fixation and a dye test have also been developed.

Control: Good management, sanitation, and prevention of contamination of food with feces. No treatment is known.

Selected references:

Dubey, J. P. 1976. A review of *Sarcocystis* of domestic animals and of other coccidia of cats and dogs. *J. Am. Vet. Med. Assoc.* 169:1061-78.

Fayer, R. 1974. Development of *Sarcocystis fusiformis* in the small intestine of the dog. *J. Parasitol.* 60:660-65.

Fayer, R., and A. J. Johnson. 1974. *Sarcocystis fusiformis:* Development of cysts in calves infected with sporocysts from dogs. *Proc. Helminthol. Soc. Wash.* 41:105-08.

Fayer, R., and R. G. Leek. 1973. Excystation of *Sarcocystis fusiformis* sporocysts from dogs. *Proc. Helminthol. Soc. Wash.* 40:294-96.

Mahrt, J. L. 1973. *Sarcocystis* in dogs and its probable transmission from cattle. *J. Parasitol.* 59:588-89.

PARASITE: *Theileria parva*, *Theileria* sp. (U.S.)

Disease: Theileriosis (bovine), East Coast fever.

Host: Cattle, water buffalo, white-tailed deer (U.S.).

Habitat: Erythrocytes, lymphocytes, histiocytes, and occasionally endothelial cells.

Identification: Form seen in the erythrocyte may be rod-like, oval, or comma-shaped. They are 0.5-2.0 μ. Several parasites may be seen in a single host cell. Multiplication occurs chiefly in the lymphocytes but also in endothelial cells. Multiplying forms may also be found in lymph nodes and the spleen where they are known as Koch's bodies, which may be 12 μ in diameter.

Distribution: A species of *Theileria* has been observed in white-tailed deer, cattle, and sheep in the southern U.S.; it is, however, considered to be nonpathogenic. East Coast Fever is enzootic in East, South, and Central Africa.

Life cycle: Details of the life cycle and the development of the organism in a species of *Rhipicephalus* are still unknown. Transovarian transmission does not occur.

Transmission: By the bite of infected *Rhipicephalus* spp. and *Hyalomma* spp. Transmission in the tick is trans-stadial, not transovarian.

Signs and pathogenicity: *T. parva* is highly pathogenic causing 90-100% mortality in severe outbreaks. In acute disease, the body temperature may be 104-107°F. Animals stop eating, have a serious nasal discharge, swelling of superficial lymph nodes, general weakness, emaciation, and usually die. The disease has various clinical forms; its severity depends on the strain characteristics. Incubation period after tick inoculation is as long as 25 days.

Diagnosis: Demonstration of the parasites in the erythrocytes in stained blood smears together with case history.

Control: Based on tick control and quarantine measures. Regular dipping with arsenicals or toxaphene has been shown to effectively control ticks. Chlortetracycline and oxytetracycline apparently are somewhat beneficial if given during the incubation and reaction periods.

Selected references:

Kuttler, K. L., and T. M. Craig. 1975. Isolation of a bovine *Theileria*. *Am. J. Vet. Res.* 36:323-25.

Robinson, R. M., K. L. Kuttler, J. W. Thomas, and R. G. Marburger. 1967. Theileriasis in Texas white-tailed deer. *Jour. Wildl. Management* 31:455-59.

PARASITE: *Toxoplasma gondii*

Disease: Toxoplasmosis.

Host: First reported from the gondi, a north African rodent; now reported from a wide range of mammals, birds, and man.

Habitat: A parasite found in many cell types such as neurons, endothelium, reticulum, liver parenchyma, cardiac, and muscle cells. It may also be free in the blood and peritoneal exudate.

Identification: Trophozoites are crescent-shaped or banana-shaped and about 6 x 3 μ with a round nucleus as large as 2 μ in diameter. The oocyst stage, seen only in cat feces to date, is indistinguishable from the oocysts of *Isospora bigemina*. Before sporulation *T. gondii* oocysts are spherical with a mean size of 12.5 x 11.0 μ. This organism is now considered to be a coccidium.

Distribution and importance: Found throughout North America. The importance of the disease remains obscure. Serological testing frequently reveals the disease in man and other animals. The disease is of human importance because the organism may be transferred from a pregnant woman to her offspring.

Life cycle: At present the cat is considered the definitive host, and numerous other species of mammals and birds serve as intermediate hosts. The sexual phase of the life cycle occurs in the epithelial cells of the small intestine of the cat and results in oocysts. The asexual stages develop in various cells of the body and are frequently demonstrated in brain and striated muscle cells of the intermediate host. Trophozoites in cysts or free in the flesh of animals are the prime source of infection for carnivores. Oocysts from cat feces are the source of infection for herbivores and omnivores.

Transmission: By ingestion of sporulated oocysts, by way of the placenta, or by ingestion of meat from infected animals.

Signs and pathogenicity: The zoonosis transmitted from animals to man may range from inapparent infection to an acutely fatal disease. Asymptomatic toxoplasmosis is probably the most common form of the disease. Signs of the acute form of the disease may include fever, pneumonia, hepatitis, and lymph node enlargement. Prenatal infection may result in stillbirth, abortion, hydrocephalus, mental retardation, and blindness in humans. In chronic infections cysts may be found in many organs or tissues where they may cause severe lesions.

Diagnosis: Intraperitoneal inoculation of mice is the usual diagnostic procedure. Serological tests of value are the dye test and the haemagglutination test. The complement fixation test is frequently used as an adjunct to the dye test.

Control: At present, disposal of cat feces in a sanitary manner is important. Meat eaten by man should be well cooked. Animal feed containing meat, if not commercially processed, should be cooked. For general prevention of toxoplasmosis in humans, especially pregnant women, the following should be practiced.

    1. Wash hands before eating, especially important for children.

    2. Wash hand after handling raw meat.

    3. Feed cats dry, canned, or cooked food.

    4. Dispose of cat feces daily, preferably via the toilet.

    5. Cover play pens and sand boxes when not in use.

    6. Wear garden gloves when gardening.

Pregnant women should avoid contact with cat feces.

Oocysts are resistant to detergents and alkali but are killed by ammonia, desiccation, or heating to 55°C. No satisfactory treatment is known for feline toxoplasmosis. Pyrimethamine and sulfonamides have been used with encouraging results in reducing the oocyst output.

Selected references:

Dubey, J. P. 1973. Diagnosis of feline toxoplasmosis. *Feline Practice* 3:14-17.

Dubey, J. P., N. L. Miller, and J. K. Frenkel. 1970. The *Toxoplasma gondii* life cycle in cats. *J. Am. Vet. Med. Assoc.* 157:1767-70.

Hartley, W. J., and B. L. Munday. 1974. Felidae in the dissemination of toxoplasmosis to man and other animals. *Austral. Vet. J.* 50:224-28.

Jacobs, L. 1973. New knowledge of toxoplasma and toxoplasmosis. *Adv. Parasitol.* 11:631-69.

Walls, K. W., and M. G. Schultz. 1968. Public health aspects of toxoplasmosis. *J. Am. Vet. Med. Assoc.* 153:1775-79.

PARASITE: *Trichomonas gallinae* (flagellate)

Disease: Trichomoniasis (avian).

Host: Primary host is the domestic pigeon but may be found in the chicken, turkey, and many wild birds.

Habitat: Crop, upper digestive tract.

Identification: Body ellipsoidal or pear-shaped, 5-19 μ long by 2-9 μ wide, with 4 anterior flagella. A free-trailing posterior flagellum is absent.

Distribution and importance: Widespread in birds throughout North America.

Life cycle: Reproduce by longitudinal binary fission; no cyst formation.

Transmission: In pigeons transfer from adults to squabs is via "pigeon's milk" produced in the mother's crop. Domestic fowl are probably infected by ingestion of contaminated food and water.

Signs and pathogenicity: Essentially a disease of young birds. Severity of disease seems to depend on the virulence of different trichomonad strains. Birds lose weight, stand huddled, and have ruffled feathers. Lesions in the mouth, pharynx, esophagus, and crop are small, yellowish, circumscribed caseous areas on the mucosa. As the lesions enlarge, they spread and become caseous masses.

Diagnosis: Gross observation of the mouth and throat lesions. Confirmation of the diagnosis is the demonstration of the flagellate in smears from the lesions.

Control: Elimination of infection from adults by medication. Enheptin has proved a satisfactory treatment.

Selected references:

Greiner, E. C., and W. L. Baxter. 1974. A localized epizootic of trichomoniasis in mourning doves. *J. Wildl. Dis.* 10:104-06.

Stabler, R. M. 1954. *Trichomonas gallinae;* a review. *Exp. Parasitol.* 3:368-402.

Waller, E. F. 1934. A preliminary report on trichomoniasis of pigeons. *J. Am. Vet. Med. Assoc.* 84:596-602.

PARASITE: *Tritrichomonas equi* (flagellate)

Disease: Tritrichomoniasis (equine).

Host: Horse.

Habitat: Cecum and colon.

Identification: A small flagellate 7-12 μ long with 3 anterior flagella and an undulating membrane.

Distribution and importance: Thought to be widely distributed throughout the equine population of the U.S., specifically reported from Iowa. Its importance is not adequately known.

Life cycle: Multiplication by simple fission.

Transmission: By ingestion of living trichomonads in fecal material or in contaminated food or water.

Signs and pathogenicity: The disease may be acute, subacute, or chronic and hosts are asymptomatic. Apparently, clinical signs occur when the host's general resistance is lowered. The most usual sign observed is an increase in fluid content of the large intestine accompanied by a protracted diarrhea. A severe diarrhea with anorexia, dehydration, and listlessness has been reported in acute cases. In chronic cases, a prolonged diarrhea may persist for a year or longer.

Diagnosis: Demonstration of the protozoan in feces taken directly from the rectum of the suspected host.

Control: Measures suggested are oral medication followed by good nursing and reestablishment of the normal intestinal flora. Iodochlorhydroxyquin is specifically active against this flagellate. In acute cases medication is given 5 days in a row. Diphenoxylate hydrochloride may be given to reduce intestinal activity especially of the colon. It is an expensive chemical and is administered in the feed. To reestablish the intestinal flora, fresh horse feces should be available for ingestion.

Selected references:

Laufenstein-Duffy, H. 1969. Equine intestinal trichomoniasis. *J. Am. Vet. Med. Assoc.* 155:1835-40.

PARASITE: *Tritrichomonas foetus* (flagellate)

Disease: Tritrichomoniasis (bovine).

Host: Cattle, possibly pig.

Habitat: Preferred location in the bull is the preputial cavity. In the cow the protozoan may be found throughout the genital tract.

Identification: Spindle to pear-shaped and up to 25 μ long by 3-15 μ wide. Actively motile showing a vigorous, jerky motion of no particular pattern. Four anterior flagella are present, and one of these extends posteriorly along the edge of the undulating membrane and posteriorly as a free flagellum.

Distribution and importance: Widely distributed throughout North America, of importance in beef cattle in the Rocky Mountain states. In dairy cattle, the economic import results from interference with the normal breeding cycle and loss of milk production.

Life cycle: Multiplication by simple binary fission. No encysted forms have been observed.

Transmission: Usually transmitted during copulation. May also be transmitted by artificial insemination and the use of contaminated equipment in examination of the genitalia.

Signs and pathogenicity: The male seldom shows any clinical manifestations other than a balanitis, painful micturition, and a disinclination to serve the female. An infected bull may be a permanent source of infection unless treated; however, the infection does not affect fertility or the viability of the sperm.

In the female the initial sign is a vaginitis of varying intensity, often with a mucopurulent discharge. In the vagina the trichomonad population reaches a maximum about 14-18 days after service by the infected bull. Even though infected, the female may conceive and give birth to a calf, but this is unusual. A placentitis frequently occurs, and ultimately the fetus dies and is aborted 8-16 weeks post-infection. Maceration of the fetus without abortion may occur.

Diagnosis: A positive diagnosis depends upon demonstration of living, motile *T. foetus* in the genital exudate of the adult or in the stomach or placental fluids of the fetus. History of early abortions, increased return service, and failure of animals to conceive suggest infection. Direct microscopic examination of washings or discharges from suspected animals may be supplemented by culture of these fluids in artificial media. Several examinations should be made before an animal is declared free of infection. A bull may be declared free only after 6 weekly negative examinations. Breeding a suspect bull to a virgin heifer will test his freedom from infection.

Control: Artificial insemination has proved an important control measure. In cows the infection is self-limiting; thus breeding rest for 3 months will usually clear up the infection.

Because bulls are permanently infected, it is necessary to treat them. Epidural anaesthesia or pudendal nerve block is followed by application and massage of the penis for 15-20 minutes with trypaflavine and surfen ointment. Treatment is repeated at 10-14 day intervals. Thorough application is extremely important. Intravenous injection of dimetridazole has been used with good results. Trichomonads may or may not survive in frozen semen in the presence of glycerol. Survival varies with different media. '

Selected references:

Fitzgerald P. R., A. E. Johnson, and D. M. Hammond. 1963. Treatment of genital trichomoniasis in bulls. *J. Am. Vet. Med. Assoc.* 143:259-62.

Johnson, A. E. 1964. Incidence and diagnosis of trichomoniasis in western beef bulls. *J. Am. Vet. Med. Assoc.* 145:1007-10.

McLoughlin, D. K. 1965. Dimetridazole, a systemic treatment for bovine venereal trichomoniasis. I. Oral administration. *J. Parasitol.* 51:835-36.

————. 1970. Dimetridazole, a systemic treatment for bovine venereal trichomoniasis. III. Trials with cows. *J. Parasitol.* 56:39-40.

Todorovic, R., and S. H. McNutt. 1967. Diagnosis of *Trichomonas foetus* infection in bulls. *Am. J. Vet. Res.* 28:1581-90.

PARASITE: *Tritrichomonas suis* (nasal trichomonad)

Disease: Tritrichomoniasis (porcine).

Host: Pig.

Habitat: Nasal cavity, stomach, cecum, and occasionally small intestine.

Identification: Elongate, spindle-shaped, and sometimes round; 3 anterior flagella and an undulating membrane extending as a posterior free flagellum. The organism is about 11 μ long by 4 μ wide.

Distribution and importance: Widely distributed where hogs are raised, especially throughout the midwestern U.S. Generally not considered of much economic import. *T. suis* has been shown to cause abortion on experimental infection of heifers. Relationship of *T. suis* and *T. foetus* requires further study and clarification.

Life cycle: Multiplication by binary fission.

Transmission: Assumed to be by close contact of individuals or possibly by contact with very fresh contaminated droppings.

Signs and pathogenicity: Although considered to be nonpathogenic for the pig, in heifers an abortion may occur if *T. suis* is introduced experimentally into the reproductive tract. No lesions occur in the nasal passages of infected swine. It is possible that *T. foetus* and *suis* may have had a common origin and are strains of the same organism.

Diagnosis: By demonstration of the trichomonad from nasal washings or culture in artificial media as for *T. foetus*.

Control: Not of sufficient concern to warrant control.

Selected references:

Buttrey, B. W. 1956. A morphological description of a *Tritrichomonas* from the nasal cavity of swine. *J. Protozool.* 3:8-13.

Switzer, W. P. 1951. Atrophic rhinitis and trichomonads. *Vet. Med.* 46:478-81.

PARASITE: *Trypanosoma cruzi* (hemoflagellate)

Disease: Trypanosomiasis (American), Chaga's disease.

Host: Primary host is man. Many small mammals serve as reservoir hosts including the dog, cat, guinea pig, bat, house rat, cotton rat, fox, opossum, and armadillo.

Habitat: Early in the course of infection, the organism is found in the blood. Later the trypomastigotes (trypanosome forms) invade the cells of the reticulo-endothelial system in the heart, striated muscles, and other tissues.

Identification: Forms in the blood may be 20 μ long with a curved, stumpy body and a moderately well developed undulating membrane.

Distribution and importance: Found in specific localities throughout the southern United States; currently not of major importance in domestic mammals in the U.S. However, they may carry the infection, and the trypanosome may be carried to human dwellings where the vectors (reduviid bugs) are established.

Life cycle: The trypomastigote is found in the blood and in the cells of the reticulo-endothelial system where they multiply to form cyst-like nests of parasites. The vectors of *T. cruzi* are the kissing or conenose bugs, which are bloodsucking members of several genera of the hemipteran family Reduviidae. The trypanosome is ingested and multiplies in the gut of the vector.

Transmission: Usually by contaminated fecal material from infected vectors. Infection occurs when the conjunctiva, mucous membranes, or skin abrasions are contaminated with fresh feces from the infected bugs.

Signs and pathogenicity: This organism may cause an acute or chronic disease in laboratory animals. Farm animals and reservoir hosts do not show serious signs of disease. The usual course is low-grade, long-term infection. In dogs general debility, anemia, and splenomegaly may occur.

Diagnosis: In the acute form of the disease, the organism can be found in thick blood smears. Xenodiagnosis, feeding by a susceptible vector and demonstration of the trypanosome in the gut of the vector, is the preferred diagnostic procedure. Inoculation of laboratory animals may also be used.

Control: Eliminate triatomids from houses, kennels, and animal quarters. Where permitted, the use of lindane or dieldrin dusts or sprays gives good results. No satisfactory drug is known for the treatment of canine trypanosomiasis.

Selected references:

Olsen, P. F., J. P. Shoemaker, H. F. Turner, and K. L. Hays. 1964. Incidence of *Try-*

panosoma cruzi in wild vectors and reservoirs in East-Central Alabama. *J. Parasitol.* 50:599-603.

Williams, G. D., L. G. Adams, R. G. Yeager, R. K. McGrath, W. K. Read, and W. R. Bilderback. 1977. Naturally occurring trypanosomiasis (Chagas' disease) in dogs. *J. Am. Vet. Med. Assoc.* 171:171-77.

PARASITE: *Trypanosoma equiperdum*

Disease: Trypanosomiasis (equine), dourine, equine syphilis, maladie du coit.

Host: Horse, ass. Several small laboratory animals are susceptible.

Habitat: Found in vaginal or preputial discharges or in the serous fluid from urticarial plaques and edematous swellings. It is a tissue parasite and rarely invades the blood.

Identification: Size 15-30 μ long with single free flagellum.

Distribution and importance: Once widespread in the U.S. The last record of the disease in the U.S. was of infected horses on an Indian reservation in Arizona. This area was released from quarantine in 1949. In 1962 a positive reactor to the complement fixation (C.F.) test was reported from California.

Life cycle: After an incubation period of 2-12 weeks to several months, characteristic signs of the disease are seen.

Transmission: Usually transmitted mechanically during coitus; organisms gain entry to the host via abrasions on the external genitalia. Horse and stable flies have been implicated as mechanical vectors.

Signs and pathogenicity: The disease is chronic, and its course may run for months or years. The genitalia are generally swollen, and a mucoid discharge is usually present. Three distinct phases of the disease are commonly seen: edema, fever, anorexia; urticarial plaques on the body; and paralysis, emaciation, death. The urticarial plaques are referred to as "dollar plaques" because the lesions look like silver dollars slipped under the skin. These lesions are pathognomonic for the disease.

Diagnosis: The organisms are seldom found in the blood. They are usually seen in genital discharge or in fluid squeezed from dollar plaques. The C.F. test is of great diagnostic value. Because dourine is the only form of trypanosomiasis in equines in the U.S., finding motile trypanosomes in fresh preparations is sufficient to warrant a thorough investigation.

Control: Destruction of all infected animals and C. F. testing of all suspected contacts. Some success in treatment has been attained with arsenic and antimony compounds and with antrycide sulfate.

Selected references:

Mohler, J. R., and H. W. Shoening. 1935. Dourine in horses. *Farmer's Bull. U.S.D.A.* 1146:1-10.

Killick-Kendrick, R. 1968. The diagnosis of trypanosomiasis of livestock: a review of current techniques. *Vet. Bul.* 38:191-97.

PARASITE: *Trypanosoma lewisi* (hemoflagellate)

Disease: Trypanosomiasis (rat).

Host: Black and brown wild rat.

Habitat: Blood and tissues.

Identification: Elongate with single flagellum attached to the body by an undulating membrane, about 25 μ long.

Distribution and importance: May be found in rats frequenting garbage dumps.

Life cycle: The rat flea *Nosopsyllus fasciatus* serves as the intermediate host. On ingestion of infected rat blood cyclical physiological changes occur in the flea, and the protozoan becomes infective in about 6 days.

Transmission: Ingestion of contaminated flea feces or the infected whole flea.

Signs and pathogenicity: Considered to be nonpathogenic in rats except nursing rats. The trypanosome may become pathogenic in rats deficient in pantothenic acid. After infection, the trypanosomes multiply rapidly for about 10 days. Then the established infection lasts a few weeks or months. A gradual decrease in numbers of trypanosomes occurs until all forms suddenly disappear from the blood and the rat loses its infection. The special immunity acquired is due to ablastin which inhibits growth and multiplication of the trypanosomes and to trypanolysin which kills the adult organisms. Both these substances are specific humoral antibodies.

Diagnosis: By the demonstration of the protozoan from a drop of fresh rat blood.

Control: Consists of flea control. Infected rats will become spontaneously cured of the infection after several weeks.

Selected references:

Molyneux, D. H. 1967. The life history of *Trypanosoma lewisi* in *Nosopsyllus fasciatus. Trans. Roy. Soc. Trop. Med. and Hyg.* 61:450.

PARASITE: *Trypanosoma theileri* (syn. *americanum*), *T. melophagium*

Disease: Trypanosomiasis (nonpathogenic form).

Host: *T. theileri:* cattle. *T. melophagium:* sheep.

Habitat: Blood, tissues.

Identification: *T. theileri:* A large species, 60-70 μ long with a prominent undulating membrane. *T. melophagium:* Similar to *T. theileri*, 50-60 μ long.

Distribution and importance: Widely distributed throughout North America.

Life cycle: Cyclical transmission occurs via the posterior station of vectors, the horse fly (*Tabanus*) for *T. theileri* and the sheep ked (*Melophagus*) for *T. melophagium*.

Transmission: Transmission is usually by contamination of the skin with insect feces containing the trypanosome or by mechanical inoculation by the infected bloodsucking insect. In the case of the sheep form, the ked may be eaten, and the trypanosome form may penetrate the buccal mucosa.

Signs and pathogenicity: Both protozoans are generally considered nonpathogenic under ordinary circumstances. However, following splenectomy or under stress the host may develop a general parasitemia.

Diagnosis: Usually demonstrable only by culture techniques but occasionally may be seen in peripheral blood.

Control: None indicated.

Selected references:

Hoare, C. A. 1972. *The trypanosomes of mammals*. Oxford and Edinburgh: Blackwell.

Levine, N. D., A. M. Watrach, S. Kantor, and H. J. Hardenbroch. 1956. A case of bovine trypanosomiasis due to *Trypanosoma theileri* in Illinois. *J. Parasitol.* 42:553.

Woo, P., M. A. Soltys, and A. C. Gillick. 1970. Trypanosomes in cattle in southern Ontario. *Can. J. Comp. Med.* 34:142-47.

PART II
HELMINTHS

Helminths

A. Nematodes

PARASITE: *Aelurostrongylus abstrusus* (Cat lungworm)

Disease: Aelurostrongylosis.

Host: Cat. Intermediate hosts are snails and slugs.

Habitat: Lung parenchyma and terminal bronchioles. Eggs are found in alveolar ducts and alveoli, often in small nodules.

Identification: Worms seldom recovered intact because they are deeply embedded in the parenchyma. Adults may be 10 mm. long; eggs are about 80 x 70 μ.

Distribution and importance: Widely distributed throughout North America; not considered of marked clinical significance.

Life cycle: Eggs hatch in the air passages, and larvae are passed in feces. After entering a mollusc, larvae become infective in about 18 days. A wide variety of snails and slugs serve as intermediate hosts; these may be eaten by transport or paratenic hosts such as rodents, frogs, lizards, and even birds. The cat is infected by eating the infected intermediate or paratenic host. The route of larval migration to the lungs is not known. The prepatent period apparently is about 6 weeks.

Transmission: By ingestion of molluscan intermediate or paratenic host.

Signs and pathogenicity: Signs are usually a chronic cough and gradual emaciation of the host. Greyish, raised subpleural nodules, 1-10 mm. in diameter, may develop. In acute cases incision of the lung may yield a milky exudate rich in eggs and larvae; in chronic infections calcified areas may be present.

Diagnosis: Identification of larvae in the feces.

Control: Prevention seems impractical because it would be necessary to keep cats from eating intermediate and paratenic hosts. Generally treatment has not been undertaken, although levamisole is claimed to be effective.

Selected references:

Hamilton, J. M. 1963. *Aelurostrongylus abstrusus* infestation of the cat. *Vet. Rec.* 75:417-22.

Schalm, O. W., G. V. Ling, and J. B. Smith. 1974. Lungworm infection in cats. *Feline Practice* 4:41-45.

Scott, D. W. 1973. Current knowledge of *Aelurostrongylus* in the cat. *Cornell Vet.* 63:483-500.

PARASITE: *Amidostomum anseris* (gizzard worm)

Disease: Amidostomiasis.

Host: Duck, goose.

Habitat: Under horny lining of the gizzard.

Identification: Slender, blood-red worms; males to 15 mm. long and females to 24 mm. long. The thin-shelled egg is about 100 x 55 μ and contains an embryo when laid. Prepatent period is approximately 40 days.

Distribution and importance: Reported from the eastern U.S. but probably is widely distributed throughout the U.S. It may be responsible for heavy mortality in breeding grounds and areas where goslings and ducklings are raised.

Life cycle: Embryonated eggs are passed by the bird. The 3rd-stage larva develops in about 2 days. After it is ingested, the larva enters the epithelium at the junction of the proventriculus and gizzard and becomes established under the horny lining of the gizzard. The prepatent period is approximately 40 days.

Transmission: Ingestion of infective (3rd-stage) larvae in food or water.

Signs and pathogenicity: A heavily infected bird loses its appetite and becomes dull, weak, listless, and emaciated. The parasites burrow into the mucous and submucous tissues of the gizzard, suck blood, and cause severe irritation, hemorrhage, and extensive necrosis of the horny lining of the gizzard. The gizzard mucosa may be riddled with galleries or tunnels containing adult worms. Adult birds do not become seriously ill but serve as carriers.

Diagnosis: Demonstration of the nematodes and typical lesions at necropsy.

Control: Wild anatids may introduce an infection to domestic flocks. Pastures and yards may become heavily contaminated. Pen rotation should be practiced. Tetramisole is the anthelmintic of choice.

Selected references:

Bunyea, H., and G. T. Creech. 1926. The pathological significance of gizzard-worm disease of geese. *N. Amer. Vet.* 7:47-48.

Leiby, P. D., and O. W. Olsen. 1965. Life history studies on nematodes of the genera

Amidostomum and *Epomidiostomum* occurring in the gizzards of waterfowl. *Proc. Helm. Soc. Wash.* 32:32-49.

PARASITE: *Ancylostoma caninum*, *A. braziliense*, *A. tubaeforme* (hookworm)

Disease: Ancylostomiasis.

Host: *A. caninum*: dog, fox, possibly man. *A. braziliense*: dog, cat, fox; cutaneous forms occur in man. *A. tubaeforme*: cat.

Habitat: Small intestine.

Identification: *A. caninum*: To 16 mm. long; grey or red depending on amount of blood in the gut of the worm. Buccal cavity has 3 pairs of conspicuous teeth. Eggs are about 60 x 40 μ and are usually laid in the 8-cell stage. Anterior end of the worm is bent dorsally. *A. braziliense*: About 10 mm. long. Eggs are about 80 x 40 μ. Buccal capsule contains 2 pairs of ventral teeth. *A. tubaeforme*: To 15 mm. in length. Eggs are about 60 x 40 μ. The 3 pairs of conspicuous ventral teeth are larger than those in *A. caninum*.

Distribution and importance: Generally distributed throughout the temperate areas of the U.S. *A. braziliense* is more prevalent in semitropical and tropical regions. Hookworms are very important helminth pathogens of the dog and cat. *A. caninum* and *A. braziliense* have been reported rarely from man, but these identifications are questionable.

Life cycle: Infection may be peroral or percutaneous. After penetrating the skin, the larvae travel rapidly via the bloodstream to the lungs and trachea. In oral infections, infective larvae usually do not migrate beyond the mucosal crypts; however, they may penetrate the buccal mucosa and migrate through the trachea. Some larvae may penetrate the wall of the intestine and make the tracheal migration, but apparently it is more usual for the larvae of *A. caninum* to enter directly the gastric glands or the glands of Lieberkühn, spend a few days in this location, and return to the lumen to mature. The life cycles of *A. braziliense* and *A. tubaeforme* seem to follow the same pattern. Whatever the mode of infection, the prepatent period is 3-4 weeks.

Transmission: Infection with *A. caninum* may be via oral, cutaneous, transplacental, or transmammary routes. *A. braziliense* and *A. tubaeforme* infections are usually acquired either orally or percutaneously.

Signs and pathogenicity: A warm weather disease of animals kept on small areas of moist ground; occurs in animals of all ages. Chief signs are anemia, hydremia, pale mucosae, weakness, and emaciation. Growth is stunted, and the hair coat becomes harsh and dry. Feces may be tarry owing to the presence of blood. Overwhelming infections in dogs are usually fatal. Blood loss resulting from *A. caninum* may be extensive. Anemia is usually caused by chronic hemorrhage; the erythrocyte count may drop to 1-2 million per cu. mm. A probable estimated daily blood loss per worm would be 0.1 ml. If iron reserves of the body are depleted, anemia soon occurs. Iron reserve depletion depends largely on the numbers of worms present and the extent of blood-letting activities of the adult worms. Little is known of the pathogenicity of *A. braziliense* and *A. tubaeforme. A. braziliense* is commonly implicated as the etiologic agent of cutaneous larva migrans (creeping eruption) in man.

Diagnosis: Clinical signs and demonstration of eggs in feces. In prenatal infection acute signs may appear before the adults begin to lay eggs.

Control: During warm weather, feces should be removed from kennels frequently. A weed burner may be used to flame the soil surface. Sodium borate (borax) broadcast over runs at a rate of 10 lb. per 100 square feet is claimed effective in killing the larvae of *A. caninum.* A salt (sodium chloride) solution may also be used. Both products damage plants. Both drying and direct sunlight are lethal to infective larvae. Several anthelmintics have proved highly effective against hookworm. Most commonly used are disophenol, bephenium, dichlorvos, and thenium compounds. Supportive measures such as a protein-rich diet, an easily assimilable iron product, and perhaps blood transfusions should be used. A vaccine prepared from x-irradiated larvae has been developed commercially but has recently been withdrawn by the manufacturer.

Selected references:

Burrows, R. B. 1962. Comparative morphology of *Ancylostoma tubaeforme* and *Ancylostoma caninum. J. Parasitol.* 48:715-18.

Miller, T. A. 1971. Vaccination against the canine hookworm diseases. *Adv. Parasitol.* 9:153-83.

Steves, F. E., J. D. Baker, V. D. Hein, and T. A. Miller. Efficacy of a hookworm (*Ancylostoma caninum*) vaccine for dogs. *J. Am. Vet. Med. Assoc.* 163:231-35.

Stone, W. M., and M. H. Girardeau. 1966. *Ancylostoma caninum* larvae present in the colostrum of a bitch. *Vet. Rec.* 79:773.

PARASITE: *Ascaridia galli, A. columbae, A. dissimilis* (intestinal roundworm)

Disease: Ascaridiasis.

Host: *A. galli:* most poultry. *A. columbae:* pigeon. *A. dissimilis:* turkey.

Habitat: Small intestine, occasionally found in the egg.

Identification: Large, thick, creamy-white worms. Males may be 8 cm. long, females to about 12 cm. *A. galli* is the largest of the 3 species. The mouth has 3 large lips. The oval eggs, about 85 x 50 μ, are smooth-shelled. They are quite similar to those of *Heterakis gallinarum*. The prepatent period is 5-6 weeks in young chicks and as long as 8 weeks in adult birds.

Distribution and importance: A very common parasite of the chicken in the U.S. Severe infections may interfere with egg production and weight gains especially in broiler birds.

Life cycle: Eggs are passed in feces, and an infective 2nd-stage larva develops in 10-20 days. On ingestion eggs containing the larvae hatch in the host's intestine; larvae enter the intestinal mucosa, reenter the lumen of the intestine, and grow to maturity in 6-8 weeks. The eggs are quite resistant to low temperatures. The earthworm may serve as a transport host for this nematode.

Transmission: Ingestion of egg containing infective 2nd-stage larva.

Signs and pathogenicity: Birds are unthrifty, weak, and emaciated; egg production drops. Diarrhea may be accompanied by anemia and intestinal obstruction in very heavy infections. Young birds are most susceptible, and heavier breeds seem more resistant than the lighter breeds such as leghorns and white minorcas.

Diagnosis: Eggs in feces or worms in the intestine on necropsy.

Control: Management is important in the control of this nematode. Young birds should be separated from old. Yards and pens should be rotated and well drained, and deep litter in pens must be kept dry. Droppings should be removed frequently. Piperazine citrate and tetramisole are highly effective treatments in water or feed.

Selected references:

Ackert, J. E. 1940. The large roundworm of chickens. *Vet. Med.* 35:106-08.

Clarkson, M. J., and M. K. Beg. 1970. The anthelmintic activity of L-tetramisole against *Ascaridia galli* and *Capillaria obsignata* in the fowl. *Vet. Rec.* 86:652-53.

Horton-Smith, C., and P. L. Long. 1956. The anthelmintic effect of three piperazine derivatives on *Ascaridia galli. Poultry Sci.* 35:606-14.

Long, P. L., and D. Wakelin. 1964. The effects of thiabendazole upon experimental infestations of *A. galli* and *C. obsignata* in the chicken. *Brit. Poul. Sci.* 5:187-92.

PARASITE: *Ascaris suum* (large intestinal roundworm)

Disease: Porcine ascariasis.

Host: Pig; occasionally found as an incidental parasite of cattle and sheep.

Habitat: Small intestine, occasionally bile ducts.

Identification: Adult females may be 40 cm. long, males about 25 cm. long with a curled, pot-hook tail. Both are stout, rigid worms with a thick cuticle. Eggs, 80 x 50 μ, have a thick albuminous coating bearing prominent projections. Female may lay 200,000 eggs per day.

Distribution and importance: Widely distributed throughout North America. Adult activity in the intestine, larval migration in the pulmonary tissues, and the condemnation of livers cause extensive annual losses.

Life cycle: Eggs are passed in the feces, and a 1st-stage larva develops in a minimum of 10 days. The larva molts within the egg to become a 2nd-stage form infective in as little as, but usually more than, 18 days. On ingestion eggs containing the infective larvae hatch, and the larvae burrow into the intestinal wall. They then travel to the liver via the hepatic-portal system, to the heart and lungs, and up the trachea; then they are swallowed. They reach the small intestine where a final molt precedes maturation. The prepatent period is 42-56 days.

Transmission: Ingestion of infective eggs with food or water or from the surface of a contaminated udder.

Signs and pathogenicity: During migration larvae may be responsible for considerable damage. Tissue destruction and hemorrhage may occur in the liver, especially around the intralobular veins. Larvae may cause numerous petechial hemorrhages in the lungs. Death due to severe lung damage may occur 6-15 days after initial infection. Adult parasites may be associated with any of the following: catarrhal enteritis, intestinal obstruction, biliary stasis owing to bile duct occlusion and resultant jaundice, and intestinal perforation with peritonitis. Young pigs are most severely affected by this parasite and may show stunted growth, diarrhea, a severe cough, and signs of pneumonia. Larvae in interlobular tissue cause eosinophilic infiltration and some thickening with varying degrees of fibrosis. These areas are a few millimeters in diameter and are often called "milk spots." Prenatal infection has not been shown to occur.

Diagnosis: Identification of eggs in the feces of older hogs, worms at necropsy, or larvae from lung lesions.

Control: Rotation of pens and runs at 10-18 day intervals, preferably every 10 days. The McLean County Swine Sanitation System should be used. Anthelmintics such as piperazine, sodium fluoride, thiabendazole, and hygromycin are effective. *A. suum* eggs may remain viable in soil for 4 years. Eggs in dry sandy soil exposed to direct sunlight are killed in a few weeks. The egg shell is impermeable to many chemicals such as sodium hypochlorite, lye, copper sulfate, and antiformin at ordinary temperatures. Boiling water is effective in destroying eggs.

Selected references:

Roberts, F. H. S. 1934. The large roundworm of pigs, *Ascaris lumbricoides*, L. 1758. Its life history in Queensland, economic importance and control. *Queensland Dept. Agr. and Stock.* Animal Health Station, Yerongpilly, Australia, Bul. No. 1: 1-81.

U.S.D.A. 1970. Preventing and controlling internal parasites of hogs. *Farmer's Bul.* No. 2240:1-35.

PARASITE: *Ascarops strongylina* (thick stomach worm)

Disease: Ascaropsiasis.

Host: Pig.

Habitat: Stomach, occasionally small intestine.

Identification: May be 2.2 cm. long. The thick-shelled eggs, about 40 x 20 μ, are embryonated when laid.

Distribution and importance: Generally throughout North America; of minor importance unless present in large numbers.

Life cycle: Eggs are swallowed by a coprophagous insect (dung beetle). Larvae develop to the infective stage in beetles. The prepatent period is about 30 days.

Transmission: Ingestion of an infected beetle or ingestion of a paratenic host.

Signs and pathogenicity: Light infections seem to cause little damage. Diffuse catarrhal enteritis and some gastric ulceration may occur.

Diagnosis: Identification of eggs in the feces or adults from the stomach on necropsy.

Control: Dry, clean lots reduce the numbers of coprophagous beetles. Sodium fluoride is effective in removing adults.

Selected references:

Alicata, J. E. 1935. Early developmental stages of nematodes occurring in swine. *U.S.D.A. Tech. Bul.* 489:1-96.

PARASITE: *Bunostomum trigonocephalum*, *Bunostomum phlebotomum* (hookworm)

Disease: Bunostomiasis.

Host: *B. trigonocephalum*: sheep, goat. *B. phlebotomum*: cattle.

Habitat: Small intestine.

Identification: *B. trigonocephalum*: To 26 mm. long; anterior end bent dorsally; mouth has large buccal capsule containing a pair of marginal, semilunar cutting plates. Eggs, 90 x 50 μ, are bluntly rounded and heavily granulated. *B. phlebotomum:* Morphologically similar to *B. trigonocephalum*. Adults may be 28 mm. long, and eggs, 105 x 40 μ, have bluntly rounded ends.

Distribution and importance: May be a serious pathogen in warm, moist temperate climates; common in the south Atlantic and south central states.

Life cycle: Eggs are deposited on the ground in feces. They hatch, and the larvae develop to 3rd-stage larvae after 5-6 days. Infective larvae may either penetrate the skin or be ingested. Skin penetration apparently is the favored method of entry. The prepatent period is 30-56 days. The life cycle of *B. phlebotomum* is similar to that of *B. trigonocephalum*.

Transmission: Cutaneous or oral entry by infective larvae.

Signs and pathogenicity: Hookworm disease of sheep and cattle is insidious. Larvae cause more serious damage than adults. Hookworms are usually more pathogenic for young stock than older animals. Urticaria and dermatitis may occur at the site of skin penetration. Young worms are associated with diarrhea, emaciation, anemia, and loss of weight in infected individuals. Adult worms are bloodsuckers.

Diagnosis: Identification of adults on necropsy, eggs in feces, or the infective larvae after cultivation of feces. Clinical signs such as anemia, bottle-jaw, and white-eye are helpful in diagnosis.

Control: Use clean, dry yards and paddocks. Stabled animals should be kept clean and dry. Wet areas should be drained. Areas around watering facilities should be concrete. Manure should be removed daily. Tetraclorethylene is still considered fairly effective. Levamisole, ruelene, thiabendazole, and trichlorfon are all claimed to be effective.

Selected references:

Belle, E. A. 1959. The effect of microenvironment on the free-living stages of *Bunostomum trigonocephalum*. Can. J. Zool. 37:289-98.

Sprent, J. F. A. 1946. Studies on the life history of *Bunostomum phlebotomum*. Parasitology 37:192-201.

PARASITE: *Capillaria aerophila* (syn. *Eucoleus aerophila*) (fox lungworm)

Disease: Capillariasis.

Host: Dog, fox.

Habitat: Trachea, bronchi, nasal cavities.

Identification: Thin, filamentous worms; may be 32 mm. long. The egg has a slight greenish tinge and a striated, somewhat netted shell. The egg is about 70 x 35 μ including polar plugs.

Distribution and importance: Generally distributed throughout North America. This parasite was quite important in the early days of fox ranching.

Life cycle: Direct. Eggs are coughed up, swallowed, and passed in the droppings. The egg becomes infective in 5-7 weeks and may remain viable in the soil longer than a year; it hatches upon ingestion, and larvae migrate to lungs in 7-10 days. The prepatent period is about 40 days.

Transmission: Ingestion of infective egg.

Signs and pathogenicity: Severe infections are accompanied by a chronic tracheitis and bronchitis. Secondary bacterial infections may cause a broncho-pneumonia which may be accompanied by severe dyspnea, a wheezing cough, and whistling noise. Open-mouthed breathing may be observed. The animal finally becomes emaciated and anemic and has a harsh, rough coat.

Diagnosis: Demonstration of eggs in feces, sputum, or nasal discharge.

Control: Keep animals off shaded soil and poorly drained areas. Use wire mesh for floors of animal pens. Strict cleanliness is necessary; no treatment is known.

Selected references:

Herman, L. H. 1967. *Capillaria aerophila* infection in a cat. *Vet. Med. Sm. Anim. Clin.* 62:466-68.

PARASITE: *Capillaria annulata, C. contorta, C. obsignata* (cropworm, stomach worm, capillary worm, capillarids)

Disease: Capillariasis.

Host: *C. annulata:* fowl, turkey, wild game birds. *C. contorta:* turkey, duck, wild game birds. *C. obsignata:* chicken, turkey.

Habitat: *C. annulata:* crop, esophagus. *C. contorta:* mouth, crop, esophagus. *C. obsignata:* small intestine.

Identification: *C. annulata:* Threadlike, slender nematodes. Males may be 25 mm. long, females, 60 mm. Eggs, about 60 x 25 μ, have 2 polar plugs. *C. contorta:* Long, slender worms. Males may be 17 mm. long, females, 60 mm. Eggs are 50 x 20 μ with 2 polar plugs. Some consider *C. annulata* and *C. contorta* to be one species. *C. obsignata:* Fine, slender nematodes. Males may be 10 mm. long and females about 14 mm. long. Eggs are 50 x 24 μ with polar plugs.

Distribution and importance: Generally distributed throughout North America. These species have become important parasites of poultry raised on deep litter. They also appear to be a problem in the commercial raising of homing pigeons.

Life cycle: Eggs of *C. annulata* develop slowly and become infective in about 1 month; a species of earthworm serves as the intermediate host. The life cycles of *C. contorta* and *C. obsignata* are thought to be direct.

Transmission: By ingesting the infected earthworm for *C. annulata*; by ingesting the egg for *C. contorta* and *C. obsignata*.

Signs and pathogenicity: Severe thickening of the crop may be caused by *C. annulata*, and malnutrition and emaciation may result. *C. contorta* is markedly pathogenic if large numbers infect an individual. Affected birds become droopy, weak, and emaciated, and mortality may be high. Birds heavily infected with *C. obsignata* may have a severe catarrhal enteritis and scattered hemorrhages. Birds lose weight steadily, may become severely emaciated, and frequently die.

Diagnosis: Demonstration of worms on necropsy or identification of eggs in feces.

Control: Control depends on the life cycle of the species and the management practice in use. For control of species with direct life cycles, contaminated bedding must be removed and destroyed. For control of a species with an indirect cycle, birds on range, should be transferred to clean ground, or earthworms should be controlled. Haloxon shows considerable promise in treatment of *C. obsignata* infections. Tetramisole is effective in food or drinking water.

Selected references:

Beech, J. A. 1967. Field trials with Haloxon against *Capillaria* in laying fowls. *Vet. Rec.* 80:195-98.

Emmel, M. W. 1939. Observations on *Capillaria contorta* in turkeys. *J. Amer. Vet. Med. Assoc.* 94:612-15.

Wehr, E. E. 1936. Earthworms as transmitters of *Capillaria annulata*, the cropworm of chickens. *N. Am. Vet.* 17:18-20.

PARASITE: *Capillaria plica* (bladder worm)

Disease: Urinary capillariasis.

Host: Dog, cat, fox.

Habitat: Urinary bladder.

Identification: This nematode may be 60 mm. long. The colorless eggs, 60 x 30 μ, have clear-cut polar plugs.

Distribution and importance: It is generally distributed throughout eastern North America. This helminth seems not to be of great veterinary importance.

Life cycle: Apparently indirect. The earthworm is considered to be the intermediate host. The prepatent period is about 60 days.

Transmission: By ingestion of infected earthworm.

Signs and pathogenicity: Appears to be relatively harmless in dogs but may be associated with a cystitis in young foxes.

Diagnosis: Demonstration of eggs in the urine.

Control: No treatment available. Rigid sanitation should be practiced, and foxes should be kept on wire mesh floors.

PARASITE: *Chabertia ovina* (large-mouthed bowel worm)

Disease: Chabertiasis.

Host: Sheep, goats, and cattle.

Habitat: Colon.

Identification: Only 1 species of veterinary importance. This is the largest nematode found in the bovine colon, and it may be about 2 cm. long. A double row of minute papillae lies around the rim of the large buccal capsule which opens antero-ventrally.

Distribution and importance: Widely distributed throughout North America especially in warm temperate regions. Clinical chabertiasis occasionally occurs in sheep but is not a major problem.

Life cycle: Infective larvae enter the mucosa of the colon, penetrate deeply, and return to the lumen in a few days. The prepatent period is about 50 days.

Transmission: Ingestion of infective, 3rd-stage larvae.

Signs and pathogenicity: Most serious effects seem to be associated with the larval stage. Heavily infected individuals may be diarrheic, passing blood and mucus. Animals lose weight and condition. Epithelial erosion, mucosal edema, and punctiform hemorrhages may occur. Adult worms feed on mucosa drawn into the buccal capsule.

Diagnosis: Finding eggs in feces and identifying 3rd-stage larvae from fecal culture.

Control: Usual parasite-control procedures for pastures, sanitation, and good nutrition. Phenothiazine and thiabendazole apparently are the most effective anthelmintics.

Selected references:

Threlkeld, W. 1948. The life history and pathogenicity of *Chabertia ovina. Va. Agr. Expt. Sta. Tech. Bul.* No. 111: 1-27.

PARASITE: *Cheilospirura hamulosa* (gizzard worm)

Disease: Cheilospiruriasis (Acuariasis).

Host: Chicken, turkey.

Habitat: Under horny lining of the gizzard.

Identification: Slender worms; males to 15 mm. long, females to 25 mm. long. The tail of male is coiled. Eggs are embryonated when laid and are approximately 25 x 40 μ.

Distribution and importance: Widely distributed throughout North America. Its importance is not known.

Life cycle: Hosts become infected by ingesting grasshoppers, weevils, or other beetles that are infected with the larvae. The prepatent period is thought to be 11-13 weeks.

Transmission: Ingestion of infected arthropod intermediate host.

Signs and pathogenicity: In heavy infections ulceration of the gizzard may occur. Parasites are in small nodules in the muscular portion of the gizzard.

Diagnosis: Demonstration of nematodes under the gizzard lining on necropsy.

Control: Confining animals to runs on bare ground may reduce infection. No satisfactory treatment is known.

PARASITE: *Cooperia curticei, C. onchophora, C. punctata, C. pectinata, C. mcmasteri*

Disease: Cooperiasis.

Host: *C. curticei* is in sheep and goat; other species are in cattle.

Habitat: Small intestine.

Identification: Relatively small worms to 10 mm. long; often reddish when fresh. The cuticle at the anterior end has a cephalic swelling. The body cuticle bears 14-16 longitudinal ridges. Transverse cuticular striations are marked in this genus. Egg size is quite variable but is generally 70-90 x 40 μ. Free-living stages are not very resistant to freezing and desiccation.

Distribution and importance: Generally prevalent in temperate climates where freezing is not prolonged. It is found in sheep throughout the U.S. but is of most importance in western states.

Life cycle: Direct; the prepatent period, 15-20 days, varies with the species.

Transmission: Via food or water.

Signs and pathogenicity: Light infections apparently are of little significance. Worms penetrate the mucosa and suck blood. In calves, failure to gain weight, emaciation, intermittent watery diarrhea, and loss of appetite are common.

Diagnosis: Identification of nematodes on necropsy. Eggs of *Cooperia* species are not readily identifiable.

Control: Thiabendazole and tetramisole are the anthelmintics of choice. Prevention is aided by good nutrition, frequent treatment, and use of feed racks and bunks, sanitary water supply and well-drained pastures. Avoid overstocking.

Selected references:

Alicata, J. E., and F. T. Lynd. 1961. Growth rate and the signs of infection in calves experimentally infected with *Cooperia punctata*. *Am. J. Vet. Res.* 22:704-07.

Brunsdon, R. V. 1966. Further studies on the effect of infestation by nematodes of the family Trichostrongylidae: an evaluation of a strategic drenching programme. *N. Z. Vet. J.* 14:77-83.

Isenstein, R. S. 1963. The life history of *Cooperia onchophora*, Ransom 1907, a nematode parasite of cattle. *J. Parasitol.* 49:235-40.

Stewart, J. B. 1954. The life history of *Cooperia punctata*, a nematode parasite of cattle. *J. Parasitol.* 940:321-27.

PARASITE: *Crenosoma vulpis* (fox lungworm)

Disease: Crenosomiasis.

Host: Fox, dog. Intermediate hosts are snails and slugs.

Habitat: Bronchi, bronchioles, and sometimes trachea.

Identification: Slender, white nematodes to 15 mm. long; viviparous. The anterior portion of the body characteristically has prominent cuticular annulations bearing small spines.

Distribution and importance: Of minor veterinary importance; a serious pathogen in the early days of fox ranching.

Life cycle: Many species of land snails and slugs such as *Helix*, *Agriolimax*, and *Arion* serve as intermediate hosts. The larva penetrates the foot of the mollusc and develops to the infective 3rd stage in about 16-17 days. The definitive host is infected by ingesting the intermediate host. The larva migrates to the lungs via the lymphatic system. The prepatent period is about 21 days.

Transmission: Ingestion of infected molluscs.

Signs and pathogenicity: Signs characteristic of a general respiratory infection such as coughing, sneezing, nasal discharge, and bronchitis appear. Ultimately emaciation and poor condition result.

Diagnosis: Finding straight-tailed larvae in the nasal discharge or feces and observing characteristic clinical signs of tracheobronchitis.

Control: Based on elimination of snail or slugs by using molluscicides, pens raised off the ground, and cages with wire floors as well as destroying vegetation near cages. Levamisole and diethyl carbamazine have been claimed to be highly effective.

Selected references:

Stockdale, P. H. G., and M. E. Smart. 1975. Treatment of crenosomiasis in dogs. *Res. Vet. Sc.* 18:178-81.

PARASITE: *Dictyocaulus arnfieldi* (lungworm)

Disease: Dictyocauliasis.

Host: Horse, mule, donkey.

Habitat: Bronchi and bronchioles.

Identification: Medium-size filariform nematode to 7 cm. long. The ellipsoidal, embryonated eggs, 80-100 by 50-60 μ, are passed in feces.

Distribution and importance: Widely distributed and seen sporadically. Of minor importance in North America; of more importance on other continents.

Life cycle: Direct. Larvae become infective about 1 week after passage in droppings. On ingestion larvae migrate via the lymph vessels to bronchi. The prepatent period is about 39 days.

Transmission: Ingestion of infective larvae from pasture or drinking water.

Signs and pathogenicity: Donkeys apparently are the natural hosts and show little sign of the disease. Horses suffer more, with severe coughing and bronchitis. The bronchial epithelium may become hyperplastic. Peribronchial infiltration with lymphocytes and polymorphs may be seen. Emphysema occurs after prolonged infections.

Diagnosis: Identification of eggs containing larvae, larvae in *fresh* feces, or adults on necropsy.

Control: Avoid wet, low-lying pasture. Separate donkeys from horses and regard *donkeys* as potential carriers. Infective larvae are susceptible to desiccation and probably do not overwinter on pasture in most areas. No satisfactory treatment is available. Levamisole should be tried.

Selected references:

Baker, D., and N. Guralp. 1957. Lungworm disease in ponies, a case report of the respiratory worm parasitism in ponies and a donkey. *Cornell Vet.* 47:456-64.

Fletcher, R. B. 1960. *Dictyocaulus arnfieldi* infestation in horses. *Vet. Rec.* 72:1171.

Holmes, J. W. H. 1960. *Dictyocaulus arnfieldi* infestation in horses. *Vet. Rec.* 72:1238.

Thomas, R. E., and L. P. Jones. 1960. Lungworm infection in the burrow. *Vet. Med.* 55:38-40.

PARASITE: *Dictyocaulus filaria* (thread lungworm of sheep), *D. viviparus* (cattle lungworm)

Disease: Dictyocauliasis.

Host: *D. filaria:* sheep, goats. *D. viviparus:* cattle, deer.

Habitat: Trachea, bronchi, and bronchioles.

Identification: *D. filaria:* To 10 cm. long; whitish and threadlike. Embryonated eggs are 115-130 x 60-65 μ when laid. Newly hatched larvae characteristically have a small cepahlic button. *D. viviparus:* To 8 cm. long; thread-like and milk white. Embryonated eggs are 82-88 x 32-38 μ when laid. The small cephalic button is not present in recently hatched larvae.

Distribution and importance: Important in temperate region with considerable annual rainfall.

Life cycle: *D. filaria:* The embryonated eggs, laid in the trachea or bronchi and coughed up, hatch en route down the intestine. Larvae become infective in 4-6 days at about 20°C. Infective larvae may survive temperatures slightly below freezing. On ingestion, infective larvae exsheath, enter the wall of the small intestine, and proceed via the lymph stream to the heart and then the lungs. They migrate through the alveoli and mature in the bronchi in about 18 days. The prepatent period is usually 32-57 days. Longevity of adult worms is variable, 56-130 days.

D. viviparus: The embryonated eggs hatch as they are carried through the intestinal tract. Larvae become infective in about 3 days at 23°C. Ingested infective larvae exsheath in the small intestine, penetrate its wall, enter the lymph vessels, and proceed to the mesenteric lymph nodes. Here they become 4th-stage larvae, enter the thoracic duct, travel to the right ventricle of the heart and the pulmonary circulation. Eventually they enter the alveoli and mature in the bronchi and trachea. The prepatent period is about 22 days. Prenatal infection is not generally thought to occur. Longevity of adults in the lung is quite variable; cattle may harbor lungworms for 6 months. The maximum life span of infective larvae on pasture in temperate climates is probably not more than 6 months.

Transmission: Ingestion of infective larvae with feed or water. Infective larvae may be ingested by earthworms and passed through the digestive tract intact. The earthworm may thus act as a transport host.

Signs and pathogenicity: In sheep a characteristic sign is persistent cough accompanied by a tenacious, mucoid nasal discharge. Animals are listless and weak, and death usually results from advanced pneumonia. Because of excessive production of exudate, the bronchi become partially occluded, and lung tissue collapses. A catarrhal bronchotracheitis with atelectasis may be observed. Pulmonary, interstitial, and compensatory emphysema may be present. Sheep lungworms do not mature in calves.

In calves and adult cattle, outbreaks of lungworm disease often result from exposure to large numbers of larvae on herbage or in drinking water. Severe coughing is characteristically accompanied by tachypnea. Mechanical blockage of the air passages is frequent as is pulmonary emphysema.

Diagnosis: Characteristic clinical signs are nasal discharge, dyspnea, and persistent coughing. Diagnosis may be based on identification of adult worms at necropsy, demonstration of larvae in the feces, or identification of embryonated eggs or larvae in the nasal discharge.

Control: First consideration should be management practices such as using clean ground, avoiding wet, marshy areas, placing animals on a highly nutritious ration, and separating older animals from young. Levamisole is claimed to be highly effective in treating sheep and cattle. In some countries the use of vaccines made from x-irradiated larvae is considered an effective immunization procedure.

Selected references:

Choquette, L. P. E. 1954. Verminous bronchitis in cattle. *Can. J. Comp. Med.* 18: 347-56.

Cornwell, R. L. 1962. Husk in cattle: Laboratory and field studies on calves vaccinated with irradiated lungworm larvae. *Vet. Rec.* 74:622-28.

Forsyth, B. A. 1966. Tramisole: A new anthelmintic for sheep. *Aust. Vet. J.* 42:412-19.

Lanier, W. 1970. Lungworm infection in cattle. *Vet. Med. Small An. Clin.* 65:801-04.

PARASITE: *Dioctophyma renale* (giant kidney worm)

Disease: Dioctophymiasis.

Host: Dog, fox, mink, and other wild carnivores.

Habitat: Kideny parenchyma; most frequently the right kidney is involved. It is also found in the abdominal cavity.

Identification: The largest parasitic nematode known. The blood-red adult may be 100 cm. long and to 1.2 cm. in diameter. The barrel-shaped egg is about 75 x 50 μ. The shell is pitted except at the poles.

Distribution and importance: Generally throughout North America. In enzootic areas it may be an important problem to mink ranchers.

Life cycle: The egg is passed in urine. If voided into water, it develops slowly in 1-7 months depending on temperature. It may remain viable for 1-5 years under optimal conditions. The egg hatches when ingested by a suitable intermediate host, a branchiobdellid oligochaete ectoparasitic on crayfish. The branchiobdellid is eaten by a northern black bullhead. The kidney worm larva is liberated in the digestive tract of the fish, migrates to the liver and mesentery, and encysts. The larva eventually develops to the infective 4th stage and awaits ingestion by the definitive host. Some investigators consider the fish only a transport host. According to Russian investigators the definitive host may also become infected by ingestion of an infected oligochaete (*Lumbriculus*). The entire life cycle from egg to adult may take as long as 2 years. It is thought that the development of infective larvae to mature females may be accomplished in 3.5-6 months. In the definitive host the infective larva penetrates the bowel wall, develops in the body cavity, and finally penetrates the kidney.

Transmission: Ingestion of infected fish or annelid.

Signs and pathogenicity: Frequently no signs of this infection are seen because one normal kidney seems to serve the needs of the host. Adult parasites in the abdominal cavity usually do not cause any marked clinical signs although various degrees of peritonitis, adhesions, and destruction of the liver parenchyma have been attributed to these worms found in the body cavity. If both kidneys are involved, renal insufficiency will probably take place. Obstruction of a ureter may occur, resulting in uremia and death.

Diagnosis: Demonstration of eggs in the urine or recovery of adult worms during an exploratory laparotomy or hysterectomy.

Control: Prevent ingestion of raw or improperly cooked fish and consumption of water containing crayfish or infected annelids. Nephrectomy may be used if only one kidney is involved. No treatment is effective.

Selected references:

Karmanova, E. M. 1961. The life cycle of the nematode, *Dioctophyma renale*, parasitic in the kidneys of carnivorous mammals and man. *Helm. Abstr.* 30:89.

————. 1964. The life cycle of *Dioctophyma renale*. *Helm. Abstr.* 33:394.

Osborne, C. A., J. B. Stevens, G. F. Hanlon, E. Rosin, and W. J. Bemrick. 1969. *Dioctophyma renale* in the dog. *J. Am. Vet. Med. Assoc.* 155:605-20.

Woodhead, A. E. 1950. Life history cycle of the giant kidney worm, *Dioctophyma renale* of man and many other animals. *Tr. Am. Micro. Soc.* 69:21-46.

PARASITE: *Dipetalonema reconditum*

Disease: Dipetalonemiasis.

Host: Dog.

Habitat: Body cavity, subcutaneous connective tissues.

Identification: Slender worms, females to 32 mm. long; males to 15 mm. long. Microfilariae from uteri are 264-278 by about 5.2 μ; some microfilariae have buttonhook tails. Microfilariae are not sheathed and have a small cephalic hook.

Distribution and importance: Distributed throughout North America; common in eastern, southeastern, and southern states.

Life cycle: Indirect. *D. reconditum* develops satisfactorily in several arthropod species such as fleas (*Ctenocephalides*), lice (*Heterodoxus*), and ticks (*Rhipicephalus*). Development of infective larvae takes about 19 days in most intermediate host species.

Transmission: Through bite of infected intermediate host.

Signs and pathogenicity: Generally not considered a pathogen. Occasional
subcutaneous abscesses and ulcerated areas have been associated with this
nematode. Because the parasite is often found in enzootic areas where *Dirofilaria immitis* is present, it is essential that the microfilariae of *Dirofilaria immitis* and *Dipetalonema reconditum* be differentiated.

Diagnosis: A differential diagnosis is most important. Differentiation is based
on length and width of the larva and shape of the anterior end and the tail.
D. reconditum larvae are usually not numerous in a fresh blood smear.
When observed alive in the blood, they show progressive movement in a
definite direction.

Control: Because no pathogenic effects are associated with this parasite, no
effort has been directed toward its prevention or control. Arthropod control should be practiced.

Selected references:

Lindsey, J. R. 1965. Identification of canine microfilariae. *J. Am. Vet. Med. Assoc.*
146:1106-14.

Newton, W. L., and W. H. Wright. 1956. The occurrence of a dog filariid other than
Dirofilaria immitis in the United States. *J. Parasitol.* 42:246-58.

Sawyer, T. K., E. F. Rubin, and R. F. Jackson. 1965. The cephalic hook in microfilariae of *Dipetalonema reconditum* in the differentiation of canine microfilariae.
Proc. Helm. Soc. Wash. 32:15-20.

PARASITE: *Dirofilaria immitis* (heartworm)

Disease: Dirofilariasis.

Host: Dog, cat, fox.

Habitat: Adults in the right ventricle of the heart and in the pulmonary artery; immature forms in subcutaneous tissues.

Identification: Long, white, filiform nematodes to 30 cm. long. The posterior
end of the male is spirally coiled and bears small lateral alae. Microfilariae
are present in blood. There appears to be a periodicity in occurrence in the
peripheral blood with peaks in the evening and early morning. Microfilariae
characteristically have a tapered head and long, slender tail. They are 270-
325 by 6.7-7.0 μ. They are not sheathed and tend to undulate in one place
on the slide.

Distribution and importance: Widely distributed throughout North America;
of considerable economic importance.

Life cycle: The mosquito intermediate hosts are species of *Aedes*, *Anopheles*,
and *Culex*. After ingestion by the mosquito, the microfilariae are found in
the insect's stomach for 24 hours. They then migrate to the Malpighian tubules where they develop and become infective during the next 15-16

days. The period of larval metamorphosis in the mosquito is at least 2 weeks and probably longer if the air temperature drops below 15.5°C. at night. After being bitten by an infected mosquito, 6-7 months may lapse before mature worms are found in the right chambers of the host's heart. Microfilariae may live for 2 years in the dog's blood and adult worms for as long as 5 years.

Transmission: Through bite of an infected mosquito.

Signs and pathogenicity: Clinical signs familiar to the owner are dyspnea and severe cough; the animal tires easily and lacks stamina in the field. Other signs recognized by the veterinarian are venous stasis with ascites and edema, acute cardiac insufficiency with heart murmur, and abdominal dropsy. Weight loss, dull hair coat, vision disturbance, and paresis of hind limbs may also be observed. The lesions seen are generally associated with circulatory distress resulting from the mechanical effects of the adult worms. Progressive endocarditis and endarteritis may occur with dilation of the right ventricle. Emboli may lodge in branches of the pulmonary artery, and areas of infarction of the lung may occur with pneumonic infiltration and consolidation. Chronic nephritis caused by microfilariae has also been reported.

Diagnosis: Identification of microfilariae of the parasite in the peripheral blood. A concentration method, such as the modified Knott's method, is recommended. Other procedures used are the direct smear, the micro-hematocrit examination, the saponin citrate procedure, and the millipore method. Microfilariae may not be found in the blood of 5-10% of infected dogs. Because *Dipetalonema reconditum* is widespread in the U.S., it is necessary to differentiate between the microfilariae of this parasite and those of *Dirofilaria immitis*.

Control: Prevention of infection may be attempted with mosquito-proof kennels, confinement of dogs in the morning and evening, and the use of insecticides and anthelmintics. Two methods of anthelmintic prevention have been shown effective. Diethylcarbamazine citrate may be given daily beginning at time of possible exposure to infected mosquitoes and continuing until 2 months after exposure ends. The dog must be free of microfilariae before treatment is begun. Another preventive measure is the use of thiacetarsamide; a 2-day treatment at 6 month intervals is recommended. It is claimed that this procedure eliminates the worms before a sufficient number have developed to cause clinical disorder. Anthelmintics effective against adults and commonly used are caparsolate sodium and arsenamide sodium. Adults may be removed by pulmonary arteriotomy in special situations.

Selected references:

A.V.M.A. Council on Veterinary Service. 1973. Procedures for the treatment and prevention of canine heartworm disease. *J. Am. Vet. Med. Assoc.* 162:660-61.

Bradley, R. E., ed. 1971. *Canine heartworm disease: the current knowledge.* Proc. 2nd Univ. of Florida symposium on canine heartworm disease, Jacksonville, Fla.

Jackson, R. F., H. C. Morgan, G. F. Otto, and W. F. Jackson. 1969. Heartworm disease in the dog—Report of a symposium. *J. Am. Vet. Med. Assoc.* 154:369-97.

Orihel, T. C. 1961. Morphology of the larval stages of *Dirofilaria immitis* in the dog. *J. Parasitol.* 47:251-62.

PARASITE: *Dracunculus insignis* (Guinea worm)

Disease: Dracunculiasis.

Host: Dog, wild carnivores such as fox, raccoon, mink, and muskrat; also reported from horse and cattle. A related species, *D. medinensis*, occurs in man.

Habitat: Subcutaneous tissues, usually of the leg.

Identification: One of the longest nematodes of man and other animals. Females may be 120 cm. long and about 1 mm. wide. The male is seldom seen and is 2-3 cm. long. Rhabditiform larvae are 500-700 μ long.

Distribution and importance: Wide distribution throughout the U.S.; an interesting parasite but not of major importance to the canine species.

Life cycle: The life cycle of *D. insignis* has not been completely described, but it is assumed that *Cyclops* is an intermediate host and that the cycle is essentially as follows: the adult female lives in the subcutaneous connective tissue and causes cutaneous swellings, papules, which become blister-like. On contact with water the papule ruptures, and the anterior end of the female protrudes releasing 1st-stage larvae into the surrounding water. These larvae must be ingested by a copepod intermediate host; many species of *Cyclops* can serve. Development of infective larvae in *Cyclops* takes 8-16 days. After ingestion of the infected copepod, the infective larvae are liberated, enter the intestinal wall of the definitive host, and go to the deep subcutaneous tissues via the lymphatics. About 1 year after infection the adult female is observed in the superficial subcutaneous tissues.

Transmission: Through ingestion of infected *Cyclops* in drinking water.

Signs and pathogenicity: Apart from urticaria and the possibility of formation of a slightly ulcerated area where the female worm surfaces, no lesions occur.

Diagnosis: Direct observation of the nematode lying under the superficial layers of the skin and identification of the nematode after extraction.

Control: Infection may be prevented by ensuring that the water supply is free of *Cyclops.* No effective treatment is known other than mechanical removal of the worm or its surgical extirpation.

Selected references:

Benbrook, E. A. 1940. The occurrence of the Guinea worm, *Dracunculus medinensis,* in a dog and in a mink, with a review of this parasitism. *J. Am. Vet. Med. Assoc.* 96:260-63.

Ewing, S. A., and C. M. Hibbs. 1966. *Dracunculus insignis* in dogs and wild carnivores in the Great Plains. *Am. Mid. Nat.* 76:515-19.

Medway, W., and E. J. L. Soulsby. 1966. A probable case of *Dracunculus medinensis* Gallandant, 1773, in a dog in Pennsylvania. *J. Am. Vet. Med. Assoc.* 149:176-77.

PARASITE: *Elaeophora schneideri* (arterial worm)

Disease: Elaeophoriasis.

Host: Sheep, goat, and deer.

Habitat: Adult worms usually found in arteries supplying the area of the lesions. Carotid, maxillary, and brachial arteries are affected anteriorly and the iliac, tibial, and digital arteries, posteriorly.

Identification: Adults to 12 cm. long; tail of the male tightly coiled. Worms frequently are found in pairs within the artery. Microfilariae are about 270 μ long; they are not sheathed.

Distribution and importance: New Mexico, Arizona, and possibly Colorado and Utah; often seen in sheep grazed at altitudes about 6,000 feet.

Life cycle: Unknown.

Transmission: Not known. A biting fly is a likely possibility.

Signs and pathogenicity: Adult worms cause little serious damage though thrombi may form. Microfilariae cause an intense dermatitis often over the head and face. Animals scratch and rub; the infected area may become lacerated. Lesions are usually 5-10 cm. in diameter and often are found over the poll. Microfilariae in lesions are periodically quiescent, alternating with periods of activity. Eventually lesions will resolve, and healing will occur.

Diagnosis: Usually accomplished by the demonstration of microfilariae from a piece of macerated infected skin.

Control: Fly control when feasible. Piperazine hexahydrate and trolene have been suggested for treatment.

Selected references:

Douglas, J. R., D. R. Cordy, and G. M. Spurlock. 1954. *Elaeophora schneideri* Wehr and Dikmans, 1935, in California sheep. *Cornell Vet.* 44:252-58.

Hibler, C. P., and J. L. Adcock. 1968. Redescription of *Elaeophora schneideri* Wehr and Dikmans, 1935 (Nematoda: Filarioidea). *J. Parasitol.* 54:1095-98.

Kemper, H. E. 1957. Filarial dermatosis of sheep. *J. Am. Vet. Med. Assoc.* 130:220-24.

PARASITE: *Filaroides osleri, F. milksi, F. hirthi* (tracheal worm)

Disease: Filaroidiasis.

Host: Dog, coyote, mink, cat.

Habitat: *F. osleri* is found under the tracheal and bronchial mucosae, frequently in small nodules. *F. milksi* is more usually found throughout lung parenchyma. *F. hirthi* is found beneath the pleura and throughout the lung parenchyma.

Identification: Slender nematodes to 15 mm. long. The thin-shelled eggs are about 80 x 50 μ and contain larvae when laid. Larvae characteristically have short, S-shaped tails. *F. hirthi* is smaller than the other species.

Distribution and importance: *F. osleri* is widely distributed throughout North America, but *F. milksi* appears to be quite limited in distribution. *F. hirthi* reported from New York only.

Life cycle: Not completely elucidated. The life cycle probably involves a molluscan intermediate host. However, there is evidence of direct transmission as well.

Transmission: Not fully understood.

Signs and pathogenicity: *F. osleri* causes a chronic parasitic disease; the usual signs are dyspnea and severe, rasping cough after exercise. With increased coughing a chronic tracheobronchitis develops, and the animal becomes more and more emaciated. Polypoid or sessile tumors may develop at the bifurcation of the trachea. They are greyish-pink and may be 2 cm. in diameter. Immature and adult worms are within the nodule. *F. milksi* occurs in the lung parenchyma and is usually discovered only on necropsy because the infection is frequently asymptomatic. Adult worms provoke little host reaction; larvae cause small, miliary, white nodules to form. *F. hirthi* is associated with a focal granulomatous reaction.

Diagnosis: Detection of nodules with a bronchoscope. Washings from the end of the bronchoscope may yield larvae for identification. Thoracic radiography may also be a useful diagnostic aid.

Control: Because the life cycle has not been completely described, the appropriate control methods are not known. General sanitation and frequent disposal of feces in kennels and runs are always recommended. Mollusc control with copper sulfate might also be considered. Levamisole has been shown experimentally to be effective in treating parasitic tracheobronchitis in dogs.

Selected references:

Darke, P. G. G. 1976. Use of levamisole in the treatment of parasitic tracheobronchitis in the dog. *Vet. Rec.* 99:293-94.

Georgi, J. R., and R. C. Anderson. 1975. *Filaroides hirthi* sp. n. (Nematoda: Metastrongyloidea) from the lung of the dog. *J. Parasitol.* 61:337-39.

Hirth, R. S., and G. H. Holtendorf. 1973. Lesions produced by a new lungworm in beagle dogs. *Vet. Pathol.* 10:385-407.

Mills, J. H. L. 1967. Filaroidiasis in the dog: a review. *J. Sm. An. Practice* 8:37-43.

Mills, J. H. L., and S. W. Nielsen. 1966. Canine *Filaroides osleri* and *Filaroides milksi* infection. *J. Am. Vet. Med. Assoc.* 149:56-63.

PARASITE: *Gongylonema pulchrum* (gullet worm)

Disease: Gongylonemiasis.

Host: Mainly sheep, goat, and pig; has been reported from a variety of hosts including man.

Habitat: Esophagus; lies in zigzag fashion in mucosa and submucosa.

Identification: Anterior end of worm has a number of round or oval cuticular plaques irregularly arranged in longitudinal rows. Overall length may be 14.5 cm., and eggs are about 60 x 30 μ.

Distribution and importance: Generally throughout North America, more commonly seen in the southern regions of the continent. It is of some economic importance owing to condemnation of esophagi that could otherwise be used for sausage casings.

Life cycle: Eggs in feces hatch after ingestion by a coprophagous beetle of the genera *Aphodius*, *Onthophagus*, and others. The definitive host is infected by ingesting the infected beetle. Route of migration to the esophagus is not fully described. The larvae probably excyst in the stomach and migrate toward the oral cavity, finally reaching the wall of the esophagus.

Transmission: Ingestion of infected beetle.

Signs and pathogenicity: Generally considered a nonpathogen; may be associated with a chronic esophagitis.

Diagnosis: Gross observation in oral mucosa. It may be seen on necropsy lying in zigzag pattern in the mucosa and submucosa; the worm appears to be "stitched" into the tissue.

Control: Use of dry, well-drained, bare lots or pens and yards with concrete floors. No treatment is recommended.

Selected references:

Zinter, D. E., and G. Migaki. 1970. *Gongylonema pulchrum* in tongues of slaughtered pigs. *J. Am. Vet. Med. Assoc.* 157:301-03.

PARASITE: *Habronema muscae, H. microstoma, H. megastoma* (syn. *Draschia megastoma*) (stomach worm of horses)

Disease: Habronemiasis, gastric and cutaneous.

Host: Equine species.

Habitat: *H. muscae* and *H. microstoma* found on the stomach mucosa under a thick layer of mucus. *H. megastoma* is associated with tumors of the gastric mucosa.

Identification: Adult worms, to 25 mm. long, are whitish. *H. muscae* lays an egg containing a larva; *H. microstoma* and *H. megastoma* lay larvae.

Distribution and importance: Infections tend to be seasonal because the activity of the intermediate hosts is seasonal. Distributions are undescribed. These species are of limited economic importance in North America.

Life cycle: *Habronema* larvae passed in feces are ingested by anthomyid (house or stable) fly maggots developing in manure or decaying organic material. Worms become 3rd-stage infective larvae in pupal and adult flies.

Transmission: Infected flies deposit larvae on the lips or around the mouth of the horse. It may also become infected by swallowing infected dead flies that have fallen into feed or water buckets.

Signs and pathogenicity: Gastric habronemiasis is not generally considered of great significance except for its association with a chronic gastritis. *H. megastoma* may provoke a granulomatous reaction which may ultimately be the size of a hen's egg. Such tumors may interfere with the function of the pyloric sphincter and may even perforate the stomach wall, resulting in peritonitis. Cutaneous habronemiasis results from *Habronema* larvae deposited on wounds and sores. The deposited larvae will not grow to adults but are irritating. The host reaction to the irritation may be an obstinate granulomatous lesion which often regresses during the winter months.

Diagnosis: Identification of egg, but more likely the larva, in feces. Cutaneous habronemiasis can be diagnosed by demonstrating the larva from a scraping of the lesion surface.

Control: Sanitary disposal of feces, fly control, elimination of fly breeding places, and stacking of manure to heat. Suggested treatment of adults is gastric lavage with 8-10 liters of 2% sodium bicarbonate followed by carbon disulfide. Numerous treatments for cutaneous habronemiasis are available. Protection of wounds is essential. Georgi suggests application of a mixture of 85 parts glycerine, 5 parts phenol, and 10 parts oil of tar. Freezing lesions with ethyl chloride is claimed to be effective. Three or four treatments over a period of 8-10 days are suggested. During the winter, lesions may be removed surgically.

Selected references:

Drudge, J. H., E. T. Lyons, and T. W. Swerczek. 1974. Critical tests and safety studies on a levamisole-piperazine mixture as an anthelmintic in the horse. *Am. J. Vet. Res.* 35:67-72.

Georgi, J. 1969. *Parasitology for veterinarians.* Philadelphia: Saunders. Pp. 184-86.

Wheat, J. D. 1961. Treatment of equine summer sores with a systemic insecticide. *Vet. Med.* 56:477-78.

PARASITE: *Haemonchus contortus, H. placei* (stomach worm, twisted wireworm, barber-pole worm)

Disease: Haemonchosis.

Host: *H. contortus* is found primarily in sheep and goats, occasionally in cattle. *H. placei* is found primarily in cattle. Sheep may also be infected. *H. contortus* does not readily become established in cattle.

Habitat: Abomasum.

Identification: May be 30 mm. long. The male is evenly reddish. The spiral winding of white ovaries around the red intestine creates a barber-pole effect in the female. The buccal cavity contains a small dorsal lancet. The male bursa has a characteristic asymmetric dorsal ray. Eggs are 65-80 x 40-45 μ.

Distribution and importance: Prevalent throughout North America, especially in the wetter, warmer regions of the continent. *Haemonchus* is an important parasite of sheep and domestic ruminants in temperate regions.

Life cycle: Eggs hatch on the ground, and larvae become infective in 4-6 days. Infective larvae are not very resistant to extremes in temperature or to desiccation. It is unlikely that larvae overwinter on pasture. The prepatent period is about 15 days for *H. contortus* and 28 days for *H. placei*.

Transmission: Ingestion of infective larvae with food or water.

Signs and pathogenicity: Major clinical sign is anemia. In severe infections in lambs anemia develops rapidly, and animals die showing few signs other than anemia or hydremia. In chronic cases the anemia is accompanied by edema under the jaw and along the ventral aspect of the abdomen. The skin is pale, the wool may fall out in patches, diarrhea may alternate with constipation, and appetite is variable. Shortly before death, animals may become weak and prostrate. At necropsy, pale mucosae, watery blood, ascites, hydrothorax, and cachexia are the classical gross signs. Minute petechiae on the abomasal mucosa result from the "bite" marks of the adult worms.

Diagnosis: A dead or dying lamb is usually available for necropsy. Adult worms may be identified on gross examination.

Control: Best accomplished by providing good nutrition and adequate mineral supply. Overstocking and wet pastures should be avoided. Use of hay racks, raised troughs, and pasture rotation will help reduce infection. Regular treatment is necessary to control this pathogen. Copper sulfate, phenothiazine, thiabendazole, haloxon, and tetramisole are efficacious.

Selected references:

Bremmer, K. C. 1956. The parasitic life cycle of *Haemonchus placei. Aust. J. Zool.* 4:146-51.

Herlich, H., D. A. Porter, and R. A. Knight. 1958. A study of *Haemonchus* in cattle and sheep. *Am. J. Vet. Res.* 19:866-72.

Roberts, F. H. S., H. N. Turner, and M. McKevett. 1954. On the specific distinctness of the ovine and bovine "strains" of *H. contortus. Aust. J. Zool.* 2:275-95.

PARASITE: *Heterakis gallinarum* (cecal worm)

Disease: Heterakiasis.

Host: Chicken, turkey, wild birds.

Habitat: Ceca; most adult worms are usually found in the tip of the blind end of the cecum.

Identification: Small, creamy-white worms; males may be 13 mm. long and females, 15 mm. long. Esophagus has a muscular posterior bulb. The oval egg has a fairly thick, smooth shell; the egg contains an unsegmented zygote when laid and is 70 x 40 μ.

Distribution and importance: Generally found in birds throughout North America. Most important is its role as a vector of *Histomonas meleagridis*, the cause of infectious enterohepatitis (blackhead) in gallinaceous birds (See *H. meleagridis*).

Life cycle: Eggs develop on the ground and reach the infective stage in about 14 days. Infective eggs are quite resistant to extreme environmental conditions. After ingestion of the infective egg, the larva hatches in the intestine in 1-2 hours, enters the glandular epithelium of the ceca for 2-5 days, and then continues growth in the lumen of the ceca.

Transmission: Ingestion of an infective *Heterakis* egg or an earthworm, a common transport host for infective eggs.

Signs and pathogenicity: In domestic fowl the adult worm is not generally considered a pathogen. Effects of the worm are slight, and only in heavy infections may there be thickening of the cecal mucosa. In some species of wild birds a nodular typhlitis may occur.

Diagnosis: Demonstration of eggs (which must be differentiated from those of *Ascaridia*) from feces or identification of adult worms on necropsy.

Control: If birds are penned, routine removal of feces and litter is important. In game farms rotation of lots and pens should be practiced. Phenothiazine is quite effective against this nematode. Tetramisole is also highly recommended.

Selected references:

Gibbs, B. J. 1962. The occurrence of the protozoan parasite *Histomonas meleagridis* in the adult and eggs of the cecal worm *Heterakis gallinae. J. Protozool.* 9:288-93.

Kendall, S. B. 1959. The occurrence of *Histomonas meleagridis* in *Heterakis gallinae. Parasitology* 49:169-72.

PARASITE: *Hyostrongylus rubidus* (red stomach worm)

Disease: Hyostrongyliasis.

Host: Pig.

Habitat: Stomach, frequently in fundic area.

Identification: The slender worm, to 1 cm. long, is reddish when fresh. The thin-shelled egg is about 65 x 35 μ and contains a developing larva when passed in the host's feces.

Distribution and importance: Found throughout hog-raising areas; not thought to be of major importance in hog production.

Life cycle: Eggs hatch, and larvae become infective in about 7 days. The prepatent period is about 21 days.

Transmission: Ingestion of infective larvae with food or water.

Signs and pathogenicity: This helminth may be found in clinically healthy pigs. Apparently a few worms do not cause any ill effects, although some catarrhal gastritis and a hyperemic gastric mucosa may occur. In severe infections carcass emaciation may be apparent. Nodular formation may occasionally occur on the gastric mucosa. Infected animals may be extremely thirsty.

Diagnosis: Identification of eggs in feces. These may be mistaken for *Oesophagostomum* eggs.

Control: Frequent removal of feces from pens and the use of dry feeding and well-drained exercise areas. Carbon disulfide and thiabendazole are effective anthelmintics.

Selected references:

Dodd, D. C. 1960. *Hyostrongylus* and gastric ulceration in the pig. *N. Z. Vet. J.* 8: 100-03.

Porter, D. A. 1940. Experimental infection of swine with the red stomach worm, *Hyostrongylus rubidus. Proc. Helm. Soc. Wash.* 7:20-27.

PARASITE: *Metastrongylus apri* (*M. elongatus*), *M. pudendotectus* (syn. *Choerostrongylus pudendotectus*), *M. salmi* (lungworm)

Disease: Metastrongylosis.

Host: Pig, wild pig.

Habitat: Bronchi, bronchioles.

Identification: These 3 species are quite similar in general morphology. They are filiform, creamy-white worms. Females may be 58 mm. long, males about 25 mm. The embryonated eggs are 60 x 40 μ when laid.

Distribution and importance: Generally throughout North America; important as reservoirs for swine flu virus.

Life cycle: Eggs passed in feces may hatch soon or after they have been swallowed by an intermediate host. Earthworms such as *Lumbricus, Eisenia,* and *Helodrilus* may serve as intermediate hosts. Larvae develop in the blood vessels or in the walls of the esophagus and proventriculus of the earthworm. They become infective in about 10 days but may overwinter in the earthworm. Pigs become infected by ingesting infected earthworms or larvae accidentally liberated from infected earthworms. Liberated larvae live in moist soil about 2 weeks. The prepatent period is approximately 24 days.

Transmission: Ingestion of infected earthworm or infective larvae liberated in soil from dead or damaged earthworms.

Signs and pathogenicity: Mainly a disease of younger pigs. Persistent coughing with dyspnea, verminous bronchitis, and pneumonia are common signs. These may be followed by loss of condition and growth retardation.

Diagnosis: Demonstration of adults upon necropsy or identification of larvae from fresh feces.

Control: Current anthelmintic treatment is the use of levamisole. Remove hogs to a clean, well-drained lot. Using concrete floors may be advantageous if feces are disposed of frequently and regularly. Using slatted floors, if properly cleaned and managed, will help reduce infection.

Selected references:

Ledet, A. E., and J. H. Greve. 1966. Lungworm infection in Iowa swine. *J. Am. Vet. Med. Assoc.* 148:547-49.

Shope, R. E. 1941. The swing lungworm as a reservoir and intermediate host for swine influenza virus. I. *J. Exp. Med.* 74:41-47.

U.S.D.A. 1970. Preventing and controlling internal parasites of hogs. *Farmer's Bul.* No. 2240:1-33.

PARASITE: *Micronema deletrix*

Disease: Micronemiasis.

Host: This free-living nematode may become a facultative parasite in the horse.

Habitat: Brain, kidney, nasal passages.

Identification: Only the female has been observed. It has a characteristic rhabditiform esophagus. Average length is about 335 μ. The egg is about 35 x 10 μ, and usually 1 egg can be seen within the adult female. Reproduction is probably parthenogenetic.

Distribution and importance: Usually found associated with decaying humus; distribution and importance are not known in the U.S.

Life cycle: Little information available for this nematode.

Transmission: Not known.

Signs and pathogenicity: Associated with bilateral and symmetrical maxillary granulomas in the horse as well as bilateral nasal discharge and prominences over the dorsolateral aspects of the maxillae.

Diagnosis: Identification of adult nematodes from suspected nasal, brain, or kidney tissue.

Control: Not known.

Selected references:

Anderson, R. V., and W. J. Bemrick. 1965. *Micronema deletrix* n. sp., a saprophagous nematode inhabiting a nasal tumor of a horse. *Proc. Helm. Soc. Wash.* 32:74-75.

Ferris, D. H., N. D. Levine, and P. D. Beamer. 1972. *Micronema deletrix* in equine brain. *Am. J. Vet. Res.* 33:33-38.

Johnson, K. H., and D. W. Johnson. 1966. Granulomas associated with *Micronema deletrix* in the maxillae of a horse. *J. Am. Vet. Med. Assoc.* 149:155-59.

Rubin, H. L., and J. C. Woodard. 1974. Equine infection with *Micronema deletrix*. *J. Am. Vet. Med. Assoc.* 165:256-58.

PARASITE: *Muellerius capillaris* (hair lungworm)

Disease: Muelleriasis.

Host: Sheep, goat.

Habitat: Bronchioles, mostly in nodules in the lung parenchyma.

Identification: A delicate, threadlike worm to 23 mm. long. The posterior end of the male is spirally coiled. The egg is about 100 x 20 μ. The tail of the larva has an undulating tip and a dorsal spine.

Distribution and importance: Unknown, not considered of major importance in the U.S.

Life cycle: The egg develops in the lung, and the 1st-stage larva is passed in the feces. Further development occurs in a land snail of the genus *Helix* or *Succinea* or in a slug of the genus *Limax*, *Agriolimax*, or *Arion*. In the intermediate host, the 3rd-stage larva develops in several weeks depending on the temperature, age of the mollusc, and its susceptibility.

Transmission: Ingestion of infected snail or slug with herbage. Infective larvae may remain viable for 12-18 months or for the life of the intermediate host.

Signs and pathogenicity: Parasite not usually found in lambs less than 6 months old. The infected animal seldom shows any marked clinical signs. Adult worms are found in fibrous nodules in the pulmonary parenchyma. Greyish nodules, 1-2 mm. in diameter, consist of areas of hemorrhage each containing a larva surrounded by eosinophiles, giant cells, and connective tissue. Lesions may eventually calcify. Heavy infections may contribute to lowering the resistance of the infected individual.

Diagnosis: Identification of adults or larvae at necropsy. Larvae from feces or eggs and larvae from nasal discharge may also be identified.

Control: Low, moist pastures should not be used, and lambs should be separated from older stock. Satisfactory treatment has been claimed with emetine hydrochloride administered subcutaneously or intramuscularly.

Selected references:

Rose, J. H. 1958. Site of development of the lungworm *Muellerius capillaris* in experimentally infected lambs. *J. Comp. Path. and Thera.* 68:359-62.

————. 1959. Experimental infection of lambs with *Muellerius capillaris*. *J. Comp. Path. and Thera.* 69:414-22.

PARASITE: *Nematodirus spathiger, N. filicollis, N. helvetianus* (thread-necked strongyle)

Disease: Nematodiriasis.

Host: *N. spathiger:* sheep, goat. *N. filicollis:* sheep, goat. *N. helvetianus:* cattle.

Habitat: Small intestine.

Identification: Very slender filiform worms; relatively long, to 25 mm. Cuticle of anterior end is usually distinctly inflated. Anterior end is often twisted and thinner than the posterior portion. Egg is large, about 200 x 98 μ, usually in the 8-cell morula stage when passed by the host.

Distribution and importance: Widely distributed but seldom primary pathogens.

Life cycle: In general the first 2 larval molts take place within the egg shell, and usually 2-4 weeks or more are required for larvae to become infective. The 3rd-stage larva may remain inside the egg for a long period before hatching and may even pass the winter here. Eggs are quite resistant to environmental extremes. The prepatent period for every species of *Nematodirus* is less than 27 days.

Transmission: Ingestion of infective larvae with food or water.

Signs and pathogenicity: Pathogenicity seems to depend on numbers of the parasite and host resistance. *Nematodirus* infections are often light, but when heavy, serious effects may result. Scours, weight loss, and growth retardation have been attributed to this parasite as well as marked destruction of the intestinal mucosa. Primary infections are characterized by diarrhea, anorexia, dehydration, and general unthriftiness.

Diagnosis: Identification of eggs from feces or adults upon necropsy.

Control: Bephenium embonate is effective against *N. filicollis* and *N. battus*. Ruelene and bephenium hydroxynapthoate also are claimed to be effective.

Selected references:

Herlich, H. 1954. The life history of *Nematodirus* May 1920, a nematode parasitic in cattle. *J. Parasitol.* 40:60-70.

Kates, K. C., and J. H. Turner. 1955. Observations on the life cycle of *Nematodirus spathiger*, a nematode parasitic in the intestines of sheep and other ruminants. *Am. J. Vet. Res.* 16:105-15.

PARASITE: *Neoascaris vitulorum* (large roundworm)

Disease: Neoascariasis.

Host: Cattle.

Habitat: Small intestine.

Identification: Stout creamy-white worm with blunt ends and a fairly transparent cuticle. It may be 30 cm. long and about 5 mm. in diameter. The subspherical egg, 80-90 μ in diameter, has a finely pitted albuminous covering.

Distribution and importance: Widely distributed; most prevalent in warmer parts of the continent. It is claimed to be a serious parasite of calves in some countries.

Life cycle: Thought to be similar to that of *Ascaris suum*, though there are indications it may be similar to that of *Toxocara canis* in its somatic migration. Mature parasites may be found in calves during the first few weeks of life, though the prepatent period is generally considered to be about 10 weeks. Eggs become infective in about 17 days.

Transmission: Through ingestion of infective eggs. Prenatal infection is probably the most usual mode of infection. Infection may possibly occur via the transmammary route also.

Signs and pathogenicity: A pathogen mainly of young calves. Infected animals become unthrifty, lose appetite, and may show colicy signs and diarrhea. Verminous pneumonia may occur. If large numbers of infective eggs of *A. suum* are ingested by cattle, the larvae may migrate, causing liver and lung lesions. Small yellow, necrotic foci may be scattered throughout the liver tissues.

Diagnosis: Identification of eggs in the feces.

Control: Strict sanitation and the removal of treated animals to clean pastures. Piperazine is a highly effective treatment.

Selected references:

Allen, G. W. 1962. Acute typical bovine pneumonia caused by *Ascaris lumbricoides*. *Can. J. Comp. Med. and Vet. Science* 26:241-43.

Kennedy, P. C. 1954. The migration of the larvae of *Ascaris lumbricoides* in cattle and their relation to eosinophilic granulomas. *Cornell Vet.* 44:531-65.

McCraw, B. M. 1975. The development of *Ascaris suum* in calves. *Can. J. Comp. Med.* 39:354-57.

PARASITE: *Oesophagostomum columbianum, O. radiatum, O. venulosum* (nodular worm)

Disease: Oesophagostomiasis.

Hosts: *O. columbianum:* sheep, goat, antelope. *O. radiatum:* cattle. *O. venulosum:* cattle, sheep, goat, deer.

Habitat: Lower small intestine and colon.

Identification: *O. columbianum:* To 20 mm. long. The anterior end of the worm is curved dorsally and bears large cervical alae. The cuticle forms a mouth collar. External and internal leaf crowns are present. The thin-shelled egg is 80 x 40 μ. *O. radiatum:* No external leaf crown. *O. venulosum:* No lateral cervical alae. The anterior end is not curved.

Distribution and importance: Widely distributed throughout temperate regions of North America; of considerable importance to the sheep farmer. Wool and meat are lost, and nodular damage to the intestinal wall may render intestinal casings of little commercial value. Carcasses of heavily infected sheep may be markedly emaciated.

Life cycle: Larvae become infective in 6-7 days and, after ingestion, penetrate the intestinal mucosa. A fibroblastic nodule is formed, and the 4th-stage larva develops. The prepatent period is about 41 days.

Transmission: Ingestion of infective 3rd-stage larvae.

Signs and pathogenicity: Lambs and older sheep with no resistance react very little to the mucosal migration of *O. columbianum* larvae. Adult worms may be found in the intestinal lumen. In sheep previously infected and thought to be sensitized, the larvae enter the mucosae, and a local inflammatory response develops. Each larva is encapsulated, caseated, and ultimately calcified. Most encapsulated larvae do not find their way back to the intestinal lumen; numerous nodules and lesions remain in the submucosa and even on the serosal surface. Nodule formation may seriously interfere with nutrient absorption, digestion, and bowel movements. Multiple adhesions may develop. In cattle, *O. radiatum* may cause inflammation of the small and large intestinal mucosae resulting in black, fetid diarrhea and extensive nodule formation. The disease is usually severe only in young stock.

Diagnosis: Demonstration of nodules on necropsy or by digital palpation of the rectum. Larvae from the feces may be identified.

Control: In colder climates pastures should be free of infective larvae after winter. Sheep should be treated to remove adult worms in the fall, late winter, or early spring before being turned out to pasture. Phenothiazine, thiabendazole, and levamisol are among the currently recommended anthelmintics.

Selected references:

Andrews, J. S., and J. F. Maldonado. 1941. The life history of *Oesophagostomum radiatum*, the common nodule worm of cattle. *Puerto Rico Agr. Expt. Sta. Bul.* No. 2:1-14.

Becklund, W. W. 1958. Bovine oesophagostomiasis. *Vet. Med.* 53:103-04.

Goldberg, A. 1952. Effects of the nematode *Oesophagostomum venulosum* on sheep and goats. *J. Parasitol.* 38:35-47.

PARASITE: *Oesophagostomum dentatum, O. longicaudum, O. brevicaudum, O. georgianum* (nodular worm)

Disease: Oesophagostomiasis.

Host: Pig.

Habitat: Cecum, colon.

Identification: These species are quite similar, thus only the characteristics of *O. dentatum* will be discussed. Adults may be 15 mm. long. The anterior end bears a conspicuous external leaf crown. The thin-shelled egg is 70 x 40 μ and is usually morulated when laid. The prepatent period is about 50 days.

Distribution and importance: Generally distributed throughout North America, probably more prevalent in south Atlantic states. Heavy infections in swine from the midwestern U.S. have been reported.

Life cycle: Life cycle considered to be similar to that of *O. columbianum*. Larvae become infective in 6-7 days. Following ingestion larvae penetrate the wall of the intestine. After 5-7 days larvae return to lumen of gut and mature. The prepatent period is about 40 days.

Transmission: Ingestion of infective larvae.

Signs and pathogenicity: Many small nodules may develop in the large intestine, and a catarrhal enteritis with thickening of the bowel wall may be observed. This nematode is rarely a primary cause of death. A subacute or chronic diarrhea and decreased appetite may cause weight loss. Nodules about 1 mm. in diameter may interfere with intestinal motility. The intestines frequently are not suitable for use as sausage casings.

Diagnosis: Identitification of eggs in feces or adults on necropsy.

Control: By use of dry pastures and lots with the McLean County Swine Sanitation System. Thiabendazole, phenothiazine, piperazine, trichlorfon, and ronnel are all claimed to be highly effective against this nematode. If only skim milk is fed for 4-5 days, 98-100% of adult nodular worms are expelled.

Selected references:

Goodey, T. 1924. The anatomy of *Oesophagostomum dentatum* a nematode parasite of the pig, with observations on the structure and biology of the free-living larvae. *J. Helminthol.* 2:1-14.

Spindler, L. A. 1933. Development of the nodular worm, *Oesophagostomum longicaudum* in the pig. *J. Agr. Res.* 46:531-42.

PARASITE: *Ollulanus tricuspis* (feline trichostrongyle)

Disease: Ollulaniasis.

Host: Cat, fox, occasionally pig.

Habitat: Stomach and 1st inch of duodenum.

Identification: A minute viviparous worm; female may be 1 mm. long. It is seldom observed because it is very small. The tail of the female bears 3 or more short cusps.

Distribution and importance: Reported from cats in New Jersey, but considered to have wide distribution. It is mainly interesting as a parasitological curiosity.

Life cycle: The 3rd-stage larva develops in the uterus; it is infective when laid. The life cycle may be completed endogenously.

Transmission: Transmission from cat to cat is thought to occur by ingestion of vomitus containing infective larvae.

Signs and pathogenicity: Considered relatively nonpathogenic to cats. The adult worms enter the gastric mucosa and are associated with hypersecretion of mucus as well as catarrhal gastritis.

Diagnosis: Identification of worms in vomitus or at necropsy. Seldom is a diagnosis made in the living animal.

Control: Depends on good sanitation. There is no satisfactory treatment.

PARASITE: *Onchocerca cervicalis* (Nuchal ligament worm). *O. reticulata* is considered by some to be a synonym.

Disease: Onchocerciasis.

Host: Horse, cattle, mules.

Habitat: Ligamentum nuchae, suspensory ligament, and flexor tendons.

Identification: Long, filariform worms, usually considerably coiled. Females may be 30 cm. long but are seldom collected intact because they are difficult to extract. Males are smaller, 6-7 cm. long. Microfilariae are not sheathed, and length differs among species. They usually are 200-240 by 4-5 μ.

Distribution and importance: Widely distributed; not of great importance in temperate countries.

Life cycle: Microfilariae are found in the dermal lymph vessels, usually in the vicinity of adults, 1-2 mm. below the skin surface. There is no evidence of periodicity in microfilarial activity. Midges (*Culicoides* spp.) serve as the intermediate hosts and vectors. Infective larvae, 600-700 μ long, appear in the proboscis of the midge 24-25 days after initial infection.

Transmission: By bite of infected midge, *Culicoides* sp., and possibly of some mosquito species.

Signs and pathogenicity: Several investigators have associated *O. cervicalis* with fistulous withers and poll evil. However, in some regions many horses are infected with *Onchocerca*, but fistulous withers and poll evil are seldom encountered. Microfilariae of *O. cervicalis* have also been incriminated as the cause of periodic ophthalmia, and keratitis and iriditis have been associated with numerous microfilariae in the cornea. Primarily older horses become infected.

Diagnosis: Microfilariae may be observed in skin scrapings. Skin in the region of the lesions or the linea alba should be lightly scraped and the tissue fluids transferred to a slide for examination. A piece of skin 1 cm. square may be excised, teased in saline, and searched for unsheathed microfilariae. ·

Control: Use of screening and insecticides should be considered. Surgical intervention may be indicated. Antimosan has been recommended; two 80-ml. doses should be administered 8 days apart.

Selected references:

Rabalais, F. C., M. L. Eberhard, D. C. Ashley, and T. R. Platt. 1974. Survey for equine onchocerciasis in the midwestern United States. *Am. J. Vet. Res.* 35:125-26.

Rabalais, F. C., and C. L. Votava. 1974. Cutaneous distribution of microfilariae of *Onchocerca cervicalis* in horses. *Am. J. Vet. Res.* 35:1369-70.

Stannard, A. A., and R. M. Cello. 1975. *Onchocerca cervicalis* infection in horses from the Western United States. *Am. J. Vet. Res.* 36:1029-31.

PARASITE: *Ostertagia circumcincta, O. ostertagi* (brown stomach worm)

Disease: Ostertagiasis.

Host: *O. circumcincta* primarily in sheep and goats; *O. ostertagi* in cattle and occasionally sheep.

Habitat: Abomasum.

Identification: *O. circumcincta:* Brownish threadlike adults may be 12 mm. long. The cuticle of adult is slightly inflated and tranversely striated. Embryonated eggs are 80-100 x 40-50 μ when laid. Newly hatched larvae are characterized by a small cephalic button. *O. ostertagi:* Adults may be 9 mm. long; eggs are 80-85 x 40-45 μ. The tip of the tail in females may have a band of 3-5 annular striations.

Distribution and importance: Of considerable importance in warm, humid, temperate regions, found generally throughout North America and especially the western states.

Life cycle: Direct. After ingestion, infective larvae tend to undergo a histotrophic phase in the abomasal mucosa where they may remain for several months. The minimal prepatent period is about 17 days. Infective larvae may survive on pasture for 4 months.

Transmission: By ingesting the 3rd-stage larva.

Signs and pathogenicity: Several forms of disease exist. In one, severe chronic diarrhea, weight loss, emaciation, and death occur. Another consists of a marked abomasitis with edema, decreased serum albumin, weight loss, and death. The larvae penetrate the mucosa of the abomasum resulting in small, circular, raised areas 1-2 mm. in diameter. In severe infections emergence of many larvae may cause local sloughing of the epithelium.

Diagnosis: Identification of larvae from fecal cultures or of adults at necropsy.

Control: Consists of providing adequate nutrition, mineral supplement, and clean water. Avoid overstocking, rotate pastures, use feed bunks, and exclude animals from low pastures. Regular treatment is necessary for the control of this helminth. Effective anthelmintics include phenothiazine, thiabendazole, ruelene, haloxon, and tetramisole.

Selected references:

Brunsdon, R. V. 1968. Trichostrongyle worm infection in cattle: Ostertagiasis—effect of a field outbreak on production, with a review of the disease syndromes, problems and diagnosis and treatment. *N. Z. Vet. J.* 16:176-87.

PARASITE: *Oxyspirura mansoni* (fowl eyeworm, Manson's eyeworm)

Disease: Oxyspiruriasis.

Host: Chicken, turkey, pea-fowl, and various wild birds.

Habitat: Under nictitating membrane, in conjunctival sacs, and in nasolachrymal duct.

Identification: Colorless filiform nematode; may be about 20 mm. long. The egg, 60 x 45 μ, is embryonated when deposited.

Distribution and importance: Southern U.S.; not of major economic importance.

Life cycle: Eggs deposited in the eye of the bird are washed down the tear ducts, swallowed, and passed with the droppings. The infective egg is ingested by a cockroach. About 50 days later the larva matures. If the larva is then ingested by a bird or other susceptible host, the worm is freed in the crop and passes up the esophagus to the mouth and then up the nasolachrymal duct to the eye.

Transmission: Ingestion of infected cockroach.

Signs and pathogenicity: Birds continually scratch at infected eyes which are usually watery and inflamed. The nictitating membrane seems to be continually in motion; severe ophthalmia may develop. In some instances, no signs or lesions are seen.

Diagnosis: Detection of parasite in conjunctival sac.

Control: General sanitation and destruction of cockroaches. Remove birds to clean pens. Treatment is the removal of adult worms with fine forceps after administering a local anesthetic.

Selected references:

Sanders, D. A. 1928. Manson's eyeworm of poultry. *J. Am. Vet. Med. Assoc.* 72:568-84.

Schwabe, C. W. 1951. Studies on *Oxyspirura mansoni*, the tropical eyeworm of poultry. II. Life history. *Pacific Science* 5:18-35.

PARASITE: *Oxyuris equi* (pinworm, rectal worm)

Disease: Oxyuriasis.

Host: Horse, ass.

Habitat: Cecum, colon, and rectum; may be seen protruding from anal opening.

Identification: Young worms are white; adult worms are creamy or slate-gray with long pointed tails. Males are small, to 12 mm. long, but are not frequently seen. Females may be 100 mm. long. The esophagus is characteristically narrow in the middle with a modified posterior bulb. Eggs, 90 x 40 μ, are operculate and slightly flattened on one side.

Distribution and importance: Widespread. Rattail condition may appear if pruritus is not alleviated. This condition is of aesthetic importance to the equestrian.

Life cycle: The infective egg is ingested with food and water. Then the larva is liberated and enters mucosal crypts of ventral cecum and colon. The prepatent period is 120-150 days. The egg develops rapidly outside the host and is infective in 3-5 days.

Transmission: Ingestion of infective eggs from feed, bedding, and water.

Signs and pathogenicity: Signs are associated with rubbing the rump against solid objects to relieve pruritus. Hairs over tail head are frequently broken. Prolonged irritation causes restlessness and interrupted feeding. Loss of condition, dull hair coat, and unsightly patches of broken hairs are the usual signs. The severe pruritus is attributed to the gelatinous sticky material secreted by the ovigerous female to bind the eggs together and adhere them in masses to the anal region.

Diagnosis: Anal pruritus and broken hairs over the tail arouse suspicion. Confirmation is made by finding the characteristic eggs on microscopic examination of scotch tape impressions or scrapings from the anal surface.

Control: Change bedding frequently, and supply clean water. If the stall is thoroughly cleaned and allowed to dry for several days to a week, the eggs will be killed by desiccation. They are not resistant to freezing. Piperazine compounds are highly effective against the adult worm. Thiabendazole removes adults very effectively and may eliminate immature forms. Local pruritus may be relieved by use of mild antiseptics or anti-pruritic ointments.

Selected references:

Downing, W., P. A. Kingsbury, and J. E. N. Sloan. 1955. Critical tests with piperazine adipate in horses. *Vet. Rec.* 67:641-44.

Drudge, J. H., J. Szanto, Z. N. Wyant, and G. Elam. 1962. Critical tests on thiabenda-zole(MK-360) against parasites of the horse. *J. Parasitol.* 48(Suppl.):28.

PARASITE: *Parascaris equorum* (large intestinal roundworm, horse roundworm)

Disease: Parascariasis.

Host: Equine species.

Habitat: Small intestine, occasionally aberrant migration to bile duct.

Identification: A stout nematode to 50 cm. long. The mouth is surrounded by 3 prominent lips. The brownish egg, 90-100 μ in diameter, is subglobular and has a thick, pitted, albuminous shell.

Distribution and importance: Cosmopolitan; of most importance in foals less than 6 months old.

Life cycle: At optimal temperatures, 15-35°C., the egg may become infective (containing a 2nd-stage larva) in 9 days. On ingestion the egg hatches, and the larva penetrates the intestinal wall and then migrates via the hepatic portal system to the liver, heart, and lungs. The larva is found in the lungs about 1 week after ingestion of the infective egg. The larva is coughed up and swallowed, and it matures in 10 to 12 weeks.

Transmission: Ingestion of egg containing 2nd-stage, infective larva.

Signs and pathogenicity: Young animals chiefly affected. Clinical signs are most frequently seen in colts 2-4 months of age. Large numbers of larvae migrating through the lungs may cause coughing and elevated temperature. Adult worms are associated with a chronic catarrhal enteritis and diarrhea of varying intensity. General debility and weakness may occur. In massive intestinal infections, obstructive colic with intussusception may occur. Bile duct obstruction and perforation of the small intestine with a fatal peritonitis have been reported.

Diagnosis: Identification of characteristic eggs or worms in feces.

Control: Infection may be reduced by general sanitation and weekly collection of feces from paddocks in hot, humid weather. In dry hot weather, collections may be made at 14-day intervals. Manure should be stacked and allowed to heat or placed on arable land or pasture not used by horses. Piperazine is specifically effective against this nematode; it is highly efficacious and practically nontoxic. Thiabendazole has also been shown to be effective. Older anthelmintics used against this parasite are carbon disulfide and toluene.

Selected references:

Clark, D. T., and N. D. Conner. 1959. Field tests on the efficacy of piperazine-carbon disulfide complex in the treatment of foals for gastrointestinal parasites. *Am. J. Vet. Res.* 20:452-58.

Todd, A. C., and L. P. Doherty. 1951. Treatment of ascariasis in horses in central Kentucky. *J. Am. Vet. Med. Assoc.* 119:363-67.

Wise, W. E., J. H. Drudge, and E. T. Lyons. 1972. Controlling internal parasites of the horse. University of Kentucky.

PARASITE: *Parelaphostrongylus tenuis* (syn. *Pneumostrongylus tenuis*) (meningeal worm)

Disease: Cerebrospinal nematodiasis.

Host: Deer, moose, and occasionally sheep.

Habitat: Meninges, blood vessels of the dura, brain, and spinal cord.

Identification: The slender worm, 5-6.5 cm. long, resembles a piece of fine cotton thread.

Distribution and importance: Eastern North America; occurs where white-tailed deer and moose ranges overlap. It is an important disease of moose. It may be an erratic parasite of sheep, causing cerebrospinal nematodiasis and sometimes a fatal meningitis.

Life cycle: Larval migration route to the brain is undescribed. The female deposits eggs in the meninges; larvae reach the lungs via the bloodstream, break into alveoli, proceed via the trachea to the pharynx, and are swallowed. Larvae develop in several species of snails and slugs in the genera *Discus, Zonitiodes, Deroceras, Triodopsis, Stenotrema, Lymnaea, Arion, Anguispira,* and *Succinea.* Larvae released from snail tissue in the stomach of the deer penetrate the ventral curvature of the stomach, enter the peritoneal cavity, and reach the spinal cord in about 10 days. They develop in the dorsal horns of the cord for 20-30 days. Then they leave the neural parenchyma and mature in the subdural space. The prepatent period is about 90 days.

Transmission: Ingestion of infected snail or slug.

Signs and pathogenicity: In sheep larvae may migrate in brain and spinal cord and cause focal areas of hemorrhage. Affected sheep may become paralyzed or show marked ataxia. In deer the nematodes seem to cause little damage, and no neurological disturbance is seen. In moose subarchnoid hemorrhages and meningoencephalitis may occur. A purulent meningitis and focal encephalitis may occur in the cerebrum and cerebellum.

In abnormal hosts such as moose, wapiti, mule deer, caribou, goats, and sheep signs observed may be ataxia, lameness, stiffness, lumbar weakness, circling, and blindness.

Diagnosis: Identification of adults at necropsy or larvae in fecal cultures from deer.

Control: No treatment is effective. Disease is density-dependent and flourishes under conditions of overpopulation.

Selected references:

Anderson, R. C. 1964. Neurologic disease in moose infected experimentally with *Pneumostrongylus tenuis* from white-tailed deer. *Path. Vet.* 1:289-322.

———. 1972. The ecological relationship of meningeal worm and native Cervids in North America. *J. Wildl. Dis.* 8:304-10.

Kennedy, P. C., J. H. Whitlock, and S. J. Roberts. 1952. Neurolofilariasis, a paralytic disease of sheep: I. Introduction, symptomatology and pathology. *Cornell Vet.* 42:118-24.

PARASITE: *Pelodera strongyloides* (syn. *Rhabditis strongyloides*) (free-living, saprophytic nematode)

Disease: Peloderiasis.

Host: Dog, cattle.

Habitat: Usually found in moist, decaying, organic material such as bedding and damp soil. It may invade damaged or scarified skin and cause a severe dermatitis.

Identification: Small, delicate nematodes; females may be 1.5 mm. long and males, 1.2 mm. long. Eggs are about 60 x 35 μ, and rhabditiform larvae may be 600 μ long.

Distribution and importance: Widely distributed throughout North America; usually more common in the warmer, humid regions. It is of some importance in sporting dogs in early spring.

Life cycle: Free-living females lay undeveloped eggs. These hatch on the ground releasing rhabditiform larvae which invade superficial dermal layers.

Transmission: Contact with nematodes in wet bedding.

Signs and pathogenicity: Invasion of the superficial layers of the skin causes a mild dermatitis, usually on the underline or inner surface of the limbs. The skin may become reddened, denuded, and covered with a crusty material. Occasionally pustular erythema develops.

Diagnosis: Identification of larvae and possibly adults from superficial skin scrapings.

Control: The dermatitis will probably abate if the infected animal is kept clean and dry. Any astringent solution such as tannic or salicylic acid in alcohol should be helpful. Sponging the affected area with an insecticidal solution such as chlordane is therapeutically useful.

Selected references:

Chitwood, B. G. 1932. The association of *Rhabditis strongyloides* with dermatitis in dogs. *N. Am. Vet.* 13:35-40.

Levine, N. D., L. J. Miller, C. C. Morrill, and M. E. Mansfield. 1950. Nematode dermatitis in cattle associated with *Rhabditis. J. Am. Vet. Med. Assoc.* 116:294-96.

Rhode, E. A., J. E. Jasper, N. F. Baker, and J. R. Douglas. 1953. The occurrence of *Rhabditis* dermatitis in cattle. *N. Am. Vet.* 34:634-37.

Schwartzman, R. M. 1964. Rhabditic dermatitis in the dog. *J. Am. Vet. Med. Assoc.* 145:25-28.

PARASITE: *Physaloptera* sp.

Disease: Physalopteriasis.

Host: Dog, cat, and small carnivores.

Habitat: Stomach.

Identification: A stout, ascarid-type worm in which the cuticle forms a cephalic collarette. A preputiallike sheath may be present at the posterior end of the worm. The female is 30-40 mm. long, and the male may be 30 mm. long. The egg is about 40 by 30 μ.

Distribution and importance: Widely distributed throughout the U.S. It may be confused with a juvenile *Toxocara* or *Toxascaris* that is vomited or found in the stomach at necropsy. It is generally considered of minor importance in the dog and cat.

Life cycle: Arthropod intermediate hosts are probably beetles, crickets, and cockroaches.

Transmission: Ingestion of infected intermediate host.

Signs and pathogenicity: Attachment to the gastric mucosa may cause small areas of hemorrhage and, consequently, mucosal erosion and gastritis. It is relatively nonpathogenic.

Diagnosis: Identification of eggs in feces or worms from vomitus or at necropsy.

Control: No satisfactory treatment is known. Control of arthropod intermediate hosts, especially cockroaches and flour beetles, is recommended.

Selected references:

Hall, M. C., and M. Wigdor. 1918. A *Physaloptera* from the dog with a note on the nematode parasites of the dog in North America. *J. Am. Vet. Med. Assoc.* 53:733-44.

PARASITE: *Physocephalus sexaltus* (thick stomach worm)

Disease: Physocephaliasis.

Host: Pig, occasionally cattle and horses.

Habitat: Stomach.

Identification: Small, filiform nematodes; may be slightly red. The thick-shelled eggs are embryonated when laid and are about 35 x 17 μ.

Distribution and importance: Generally throughout the U.S.; usually not a parasite of major importance.

Life cycle: The embryonated egg is ingested by a coprophagous beetle which, in turn, may be eaten by a paratenic host. The prepatent period is about 6 weeks.

Transmission: Ingestion of infected beetle or infected paratenic host.

Signs and pathogenicity: Fundic area of the stomach may show some hyperemia with an acute or chronic gastritis. Hogs may be retarded in growth.

Diagnosis: Identification of eggs in feces or adults on necropsy.

Control: Use of clean, dry yards and pens. Anthelmintics of choice would be carbon disulfide and sodium fluoride.

PARASITE: *Probstmayria vivipara*

Disease: Probstmayriasis.

Host: Equine species.

Habitat: Colon.

Identification: A minute, viviparous nematode to 2 mm. long. Before birth the larva is almost as large as its parent. This nematode is one of the few that multiply within hosts.

Distribution and importance: Probably widely distributed but seldom seen; probably not important.

Life cycle: Multiplies without leaving its host. Populations within the host may become very large.

Transmission: Unknown, presumably by ingestion of larvae in feces.

Signs and pathogenicity: Not known to be pathogenic.

Diagnosis: Identification of adults in colon contents at necropsy.

Control: Appears to be susceptible to the broad-spectrum anthelmintics. Thiabendazole is currently the drug of choice.

Selected references:

LeRoux, P. L. 1924. Helminths collected from equines in Edinburgh and in London. *J. Helminthol.* 2:111-34.

PARASITE: *Setaria cervi* (syn. *Setaria labiato-papillosa*) (peritoneal worm, abdominal worm)

Disease: Setariasis.

Host: Cattle, deer.

Habitat: Peritoneal cavity, occasionally in other organs and tissues.

Identification: Females may be 120 mm. long; males are half as long. Microfilariae are sheathed and are about 250 x 7 μ.

Distribution and importance: Generally throughout North America; of no known economic importance in this country. Cerebrospinal nematodiasis is associated with this parasite in other countries.

Life cycle: No periodicity in microfilarial activity. Microfilariae develop in the thoracic muscles of the mosquito and, in warm climates, are infective after about 12 days in the mosquito. The prepatent period varies from 8-10 months.

Transmission: By the bite of the mosquito. In tropical countries the vectors include species of *Culex*, *Anopheles*, and *Aedes*.

Signs and pathogenicity: In temperate climates this parasite is generally nonpathogenic. In some warmer climates the nematodes invade the spinal canal of sheep and goats causing cerebrospinal meningitis which may result in paralysis and death.

Diagnosis: Demonstration of microfilariae in blood.

Control: Control is not usually attempted.

Selected references:

Becklund, W. W. 1959. Worm parasites in cattle from south Georgia. *Vet. Med.* 54: 369-72.

Yeh, L. S. 1959. A revision of the nematode genus *Setaria*, Viborg, 1795, its host-parasite relationship, speciation and evolution. *J. Helminthol.* 33:1-98.

PARASITE: *Setaria equina* (abdominal worm)

Disease: Setariasis.

Host: Equine species and occasionally cattle; intermediate host is a culicene mosquito.

Habitat: Peritoneal cavity but has been recorded from other organs and tissues such as scrotum. It is not uncommon in the eyes of cattle.

Identification: Long, slender, whitish worms. Males may be 80 mm. and females, 130 mm. long. Males usually have a characteristically spiral tail. Sheathed microfilariae are 240-256 μ long.

Distribution and importance: Widely distributed. Its importance is negligible if it is in the peritoneal cavity, but it may cause serious damage if the eye is invaded. This helminth is frequently seen at necropsy.

Life cycle: Slightly more microfilariae are found in the peripheral blood at night, especially in hosts in tropical areas. Microfilariae develop in culicine mosquitoes such as members of the genera *Aedes* and *Culex*. Depending on environmental temperature, larvae become infective in 12-16 days. The prepatent period is 8-10 months.

Transmission: Bite of infected species of *Aedes* or *Culex*.

Signs and pathogenicity: Adults in the peritoneal cavity are nonpathogenic. A slight fibrinous peritonitis may occasionally be observed.

Diagnosis: Identification of sheathed microfilariae in blood smears or adults at necropsy.

Control: Not generally attempted because it is usually nonpathogenic.

Selected references:

Schwartz, B. 1927. Nematodes belonging to the genus *Setaria* parasitic in the eyes of horses. *N. Am. Vet.* 8:24-27.

PARASITE: *Spirocerca lupi* (esophageal or gullet worm)

Disease: Spirocercosis.

Host: Dog, fox, wolf. Intermediate host is a coprophagous insect, the dung beetle.

Habitat: Wall of the esophagus and stomach. Occasionally it is free in the stomach, or it embeds in the wall of the aorta.

Identification: Worms are large, to 8 cm. long and stout. They are usually coiled and reddish when fresh. Males have a characteristic spiral posterior end. The thick-shelled eggs are 40 x 12 μ and contain larvae when laid.

Distribution and importance: Most widely distributed in southern regions of the U.S.

Life cycle: Eggs hatch only after ingestion by a suitable coprophagous beetle. Larvae become infective and encyst in the tracheal tubes of the beetle. On ingestion of the infected beetle, larvae are liberated in the stomach, penetrate the stomach wall, and find their way via the arterial system to the aorta and then to the esophagus. If eaten by an unsuitable host, the larvae may become encysted in the esophagus, mesentery, or other organs of the paratenic host (hedgehog or lizard). The prepatent period is about 5½ months.

Transmission: Ingestion of infected coprophagous beetle or paratenic host.

Signs and pathogenicity: Esophageal lesions may interfere with deglutition, respiration, and circulation. Lesions in the stomach may cause vomiting. Neoplasm development is accompanied by wasting and general emaciation. Secondary effects of spirocercosis are of considerable interest. A hypertrophic pulmonary osteoarthropathy is thought to be presumptive evidence of spirocercosis. More important is speculation that this helminth may cause malignant gastric neoplasms, usually osteosarcomas.

Diagnosis: Presence of esophageal lesions and demonstration from feces of small, elongate eggs with thick shells are helpful. However, eggs pass from lesions to the esophagus intermittently, and repeated fecal examination may be necessary to demonstrate the eggs. Tumors may be satisfactorily detected by manual palpation or x-ray examination.

Control: Isolate animals and carefully dispose of vomitus and feces. Disophenol is claimed to be therapeutically useful.

Selected references:

Bailey, W. S. 1963. Parasites and cancer; sarcoma in dogs associated with *Spirocerca lupi. Ann. N. Y. Acad. Sci.* 108:890-923.

———. 1972. *Spirocerca lupi*, a continuing inquiry. *J. Parasitol.* 58:3-22.
Darne, A., and J. L. Webb. 1964. The treatment of ankylostomiasis and of spirocercosis in dogs by the new compound, 2, 6-diiodo-4-nitrophenol. *Vet. Rec.* 76:171-72.

PARASITE: *Stephanofilaria stilesi*

Disease: Stephanofilariasis.
Host: Cattle.
Habitat: Epithelium of skin on midventral line of abdomen, especially in beef cattle.
Identification: Very small nematodes, to 8 mm. long.
Distribution and importance: Generally throughout the U.S., more common in western range and irrigated country. It is more usual in beef animals than in other cattle.
Life cycle: Transmitted by the horn fly which ingests microfilaria from lesions on the underline. Larval development in the vector takes 18-21 days. The definitive host is infected when flies bite the skin on the underline. Adult worms mature and lay eggs on the skin about 6-8 weeks after infection.
Transmission: Through bite of an infected horn fly, *Haematobia irritans*.
Signs and pathogenicity: Lesion begins as a papular dermatitis. A long-standing irritation develops, and the skin surface becomes ulcerated. Dermatitis may extend from the brisket to the umbilicus, but the abdomen, udder, scrotum, and flanks may also be involved. Signs are usually seen in animals 8-10 months old.
Diagnosis: Because microfilariae are not blood-borne, they may be observed in smears or scrapings taken from the lesion.
Controls: Use insecticides to control the horn fly. Application of disinfectant and wound-healing powder is recommended for treatment of lesions.

Selected references:
Dikmans, G. 1948. Skin lesions of domestic animals in the U.S. due to nematode infestation. *Cornell Vet.* 38:3-23.
Hibler, C. P. 1966. Development of *Stephanofilaria stilesi* in the horn fly. *J. Parasitol.* 52:890-98.
Levine, N. D., and C. C. Morrill. 1955. Bovine stephanofilarial dermatitis in Illinois. *J. Am. Vet. Med. Assoc.* 127:528-30.
Maddy, K. T. 1955. Stephanofilarial dermatitis of cattle. *N. Am. Vet.* 36:275-78.

PARASITE: *Stephanurus dentatus* (kidney worm)

Disease: Stephanurosis.
Host: Pig.

Habitat: Kidney and perirenal tissues. Occasionally it is found in the liver, spinal canal, and other organs and tissues.

Identification: The stout, creamy-white worm may be 30 by 2 mm. The adult has a thick-walled buccal capsule. The egg is about 100 x 60 μ.

Distribution and importance: South Atlantic and south central states; this parasite is usually found in tropical and subtropical regions. Condemnation and trimming of hog carcasses as unfit for human consumption cause heavy annual losses.

Life cycle: Adult worms usually found in cysts connected with the ureters. Eggs are passed in the host's urine. Larvae reach the infective stage in about 4-6 days at the optimum temperature of 26°C. Eggs and all larval stages are rapidly killed by freezing and drying. Infective larvae may live in moist surroundings for 5 months. The prepatent period is 9-16 months.

Transmission: Peroral, percutaneous, or prenatal. It may be acquired by ingestion of the earthworm, a paratenic host.

Signs and pathogenicity: General effects are depressed growth rate, loss of appetite, and emaciation. Stiffness and posterior paralysis may occur. Larvae may wander through the spleen, muscles, and other areas where they may do considerable damage. Minor lesions at the point of larval penetration may be associated with percutaneous infections. Larvae migrating through the liver may cause acutely inflamed lesions. Hepatic abscesses may occur, and liver cirrhosis is common.

Diagnosis: Identification of eggs from urine if the host is old enough to harbor an egg-laying adult; identification of worms in and around the perirenal tissues.

Control: General sanitation and use of the McLean County Swine Sanitation System are helpful. A system of biological control has proved highly satisfactory for this helminth. Kidney-worm infections may be eradicated in about 2 years by using only gilts for breeding and removing them from the premises after the pigs are weaned. Kidney worms require 9-16 months to mature and begin egg production. A gilt may thus wean her pigs and be disposed of before any kidney-worm eggs are released. By breeding only gilts, lots and pastures may be free of kidney worm after 3 or 4 farrowing seasons.

Selected references:

Batte, E. G., R. Harkema, and J. C. Osborne. 1960. Observations on the life cycle and pathogenicity of the swine kidney worm (*Stephanurus dentatus*). *J. Am. Vet. Med. Assoc.* 136:622-25.

Batte, E. G., D. J. Moncol, and C. W. Barber. 1966. Prenatal infection with the swine kidney worm (*Stephanurus dentatus*) and associated lesions. *J. Am. Vet. Med. Assoc.* 149:758-65.

Stewart, T. B., and F. G. Tromba. 1957. The control of the swine kidney worm (*Stephanurus dentatus*) through management. *J. Parasitol.* 43(Suppl.):19-20.

PARASITE: *Strongyloides papillosus* (intestinal threadworm)

Disease: Strongyloidiasis.

Host: Cattle and sheep.

Habitat: Usually upper small intestine.

Identification: Only females are seen as parasites. The small, threadlike adult may be 6 mm. long. The female is colorless and characteristically has a long esophagus and a blunt tail. The egg is small, 40-60 by 25 μ, and contains a larva when passed in the feces of herbivores.

Distribution and importance: Widely distributed especially in warm, humid areas. Young animals are most severely affected.

Life cycle: Parasitic females are parthenogenetic. The eggs are laid outside the host, and the 1st-stage larvae develop either into free-living males and females or into infective 3rd-stage larvae (filariform) which become parasitic females on entering a host. The prepatent period is 7-9 days or less. Adults probably survive only a few months.

Transmission: By skin penetration usually. If infective larvae are ingested, they penetrate the buccal or esophageal epithelium.

Signs and pathogenicity: Clinical signs such as anorexia, weight loss, and diarrhea, at necropsy erosion of intestinal mucosae has been reported from experimental studies. Young animals are most seriously affected as evidenced by loss of appetite, retarded growth, and poor condition.

Diagnosis: In ruminants, by identification of the embryonated egg from fresh feces or by identification of the larva from fecal cultures.

Control: Desiccation kills infective larvae. Clean, dry quarters and well-drained pastures are essential. Thiabendazole is claimed to be highly effective.

Selected references:

Basir, M. A. 1950. The morphology and development of the sheep nematode, *Strongyloides papillosus* (Wedl, 1856). *Can. J. Res. D.* 28:173-96.

Gaillard, H. 1967. Pathogenesis of *Strongyloides*. *Helminthol. Abstr.* 36:247-60.

Turner, J. H., and G. I. Wilson. 1958. Strongyloidiasis in lambs. *Vet. Med.* 53:242-43.

PARASITE: *Strongyloides ransomi* (intestinal threadworm)

Disease: Strongyloidiasis.

Host: Pig.

Habitat: Small intestine.

Identification: Parasitic females may be 5 mm. long and have a slender tail. Eggs are 50 x 30 μ. Free-living females are about 1 mm. long; free-living males are 850-900 μ long.

Distribution and importance: Generally found throughout North America. Only during the past decade has this nematode been considered a significant pathogen of swine. Annual loss due to mortality and morbidity is extensive, especially in the southeastern U.S.

Life cycle: The life cycle consists of both parasitic and free-living generations. Parthenogenetic females live in the mucosa of the small intestine and lay embryonated eggs. These pass out with the feces and hatch to 1st-stage, rhabditiform larvae, which may develop either directly into infective larvae or into free-living males and females that later may produce infective larvae.

Infective larvae may penetrate unbroken skin and hair follicles, or they may be ingested. If larvae enter through the skin, they migrate to the capillaries and eventually reach the lungs. After entering the air passages, they are coughed up, swallowed, and become adult parthenogenetic females in the small intestine. The prepatent period is 6-9 days. If infective larvae are ingested, it is thought they develop directly to adults in the small intestine without any migration. Development seems dependent on the environment and the strain of the parasite.

Transmission: Peroral, percutaneous, or via colostrum.

Signs and pathogenicity: A dermatitis, that may resemble sarcoptic mange, may result from larval penetration. In suckling pigs, the intestinal form of the disease may be accompanied by general unthriftiness, diarrhea, loss of weight, and a mortality as high as 50%. Piglets become listless and dull, have a poor appetite, and move very little.

Diagnosis: Identification of embryonated eggs from *fresh* feces or demonstration of female worms from mucosal scraping of the intestine on necropsy.

Control: Good sanitation, dry bedding, clean, dry lots and pastures, and use of the McLean County Swine Sanitation System are all appropriate control measures. Apparently both thiabendazole and trichlorfon are highly effective against this nematode.

Selected references:

Ames, E. R., R. B. Wescott, and J. Chang. 1973. *Strongyloides ransomi* infection in baby pigs in Missouri. *J. Am. Vet. Med. Assoc.* 163:161-62.

Batte, E. G., and D. J. Moncol. 1967. Colostral infection of newborn pigs by *Strongyloides ransomi. Vet. Med. Rev.* 272-76.

Moncol, D. J., and E. G. Batte. 1967. Porcine strongyloidiasis treatment and control. *J. Am. Vet. Med. Assoc.* 9:1177-81.

PARASITE: *Strongyloides stercoralis* var. *canis* (intestinal thread-worm)

Disease: Strongyloidiasis.

Host: Domestic carnivores and man. It is thought that each host species is parasitized by a different strain or variety.

Habitat: Small intestine.

Identification: Parasitic females are about 2 mm. long and only about 35 μ wide. Embryonated eggs are about 55 x 30 μ when laid. They hatch and develop into rhabditiform larvae before passing out in the feces. Free-living males and females are minute and have a characteristic rhabditiform esophagus. Free-living males are about 1.0 mm. long; free females are about 1.0-1.5 mm. long. Infective filariform larvae are long and slender, about 600 by 17 μ.

Distribution and importance: More prevalent in tropical and semitropic climates but also found in many temperate regions. The importance of this nematode has not been fully evaluated.

Life cycle: This nematode has both parasitic and free-living generations. The parasitic females are generally considered parthenogenetic. Their ova develop into 1st-stage larvae which may develop directly into 3rd-stage infective larvae (filariform) or may develop into free-living males and females that subsequently may produce infective larvae. The prepatent period is 5-7 days.

Transmission: Primarily by skin penetration.

Signs and pathogenicity: Dependent on numbers of worms present. If adults are very numerous, erosion of the intestinal mucosa, accompanied by diarrhea, dysentery, loss of appetite, loss of weight, listlessness, and weakness, may occur. Dehydration and death may ensue. Infections in young dogs may be very important owing to the pathogenicity of the worm.

Diagnosis: Identification of eggs containing larvae or, more commonly, larvae free in the feces.

Control: Low temperatures and desiccation may destroy the free-living and infective stages of this nematode. Thiabendazole has proved an effective anthelmintic.

Selected references:

Little, M. D. 1966. Comparative morphology of six species of *Strongyloides* and redefinition of the genus. *J. Parasitol.* 52:69-84.

Lucker, J. T. 1942. The dog Strongyloides, with special reference to occurrence and diagnosis of infections with the parasite. *Vet. Med.* 37:128-37.

PARASITE: *Strongyloides westeri* (intestinal threadworm)

Disease: Strongyloidiasis.

Host: Horse, usually foal.

Habitat: Small intestine.

Identification: Delicate slender worms as long as 9 mm. The eggs, 50 x 30 μ, are embryonated when passed in the feces. Only parasitic females have been observed.

Distribution and importance: Widespread; not considered important in adults but may be a significant pathogen in colts.

Life cycle: Parthenogenetic females produce ova. The larvae may develop directly to infective (filariform) larvae or may develop into free-living males and females. These males and females may then produce either more free-living males and females or filariform larvae. Infective larvae may penetrate the skin or may be ingested. If they penetrate the skin, the larvae migrate via the bloodstream to the lungs, are coughed up, and mature in the intestine. The prepatent period is 5-7 days.

Transmission: Infective larvae are ingested or penetrate the skin; also reported to be transmitted via mare's milk.

Signs and pathogenicity: An acute diarrhea may occur in heavily infected colts, and scouring in nursing foals has been attributed to *S. westeri*. Marked diarrhea may lead to loss of condition and emaciation. Very large numbers of worms may be found in apparently normal, healthy animals.

Diagnosis: Identification of eggs containing larvae from freshly collected feces. If feces are not fresh, both rhabditiform and filariform larvae may be observed free in the feces.

Control: Provide clean, dry quarters. Desiccation will control the free-living forms of this nematode. Thiabendazole is effective therapeutically.

Selected references:

Drudge, J. H., and E. T. Lyons. 1966. Control of internal parasites of the horse. *J. Am. Vet. Med. Assoc.* 148:378-83.

Pande, B. P., and P. Rai. 1960. The nematode genus *Strongyloides* Grassi, 1879 in Indian livestock. I. Observations on natural infections in the donkey (*Equus asinus*) *Br. Vet. J.* 116:281-83.

PARASITE: *Strongylus vulgaris, S. equinus, S. edentatus* (large strongyles, redworms, blood worms)

Disease: Strongylidosis.

Host: Equine species.

Habitat: Large intestine and cecum.

Identification: *S. vulgaris:* Brownish or reddish if blood has been ingested recently. The robust worm may be 24 mm. long; this is the smallest of the 3 species. The buccal capsule contains 2 ear-shaped, dorsal teeth at its base. The egg is 85-90 by 50 μ. *S. equinus:* The stout, reddish-black worm may be up to 50 mm. long. At the base of the buccal capsule is a large, dorsal tooth with a bifid tip and 2 smaller, subventral teeth. The oval egg is 70-85 by 45 μ. *S. edentatus:* May be 45 mm. long. The buccal capsule contains no teeth, but the dorsal gutter is well developed. The egg is 75-85 by 50 μ.

Distribution and importance: Prevalent wherever horses are found. All 3 species cause considerable economic loss; *S. vulgaris* is especially damaging.

Life cycle: Details of life cycles remain controversial for these species.

S. vulgaris: Ingested infective larvae penetrate the intestinal wall and develop to 4th-stage larvae in about 8 days. These migrate, penetrate the intima of the submucosal arterioles, and migrate in these vessels toward the anterior mesenteric artery. About 45 days after initial infection 4th-stage larvae return via the arterial system to the submucosae of the cecum and colon where they become 5th-stage larvae about 3 months after original infection. They enter the lumen, mature, and produce eggs about 180-200 days after the original infection. Some larvae remain as 4th- or 5th-stage larvae in aneurysms in the cranial mesenteric artery.

S. equinus: Larvae of this species penetrate the mucosae of the cecum and colon and migrate to the subserosa where they become enclosed in nodules. Fourth-stage larvae migrate from these nodules to the abdominal cavity and then to the liver where they may wander for several months. In the liver they molt to become 5th-stage larvae, leave the liver, and return to the large intestine. They may invade the pancreas and peritoneal cavity before moving to the lumen of the cecum and colon. After entering the colon the larvae mature, and adult worms produce eggs about 270 days after the initial infection.

S. edentatus: Infective larvae enter the wall of the intestine and reach the liver via the portal circulation. Fourth-stage larvae migrate in the liver for as long as 9 weeks. They then wander between the peritoneal layers of the hepatic ligaments to reach the parietal peritoneum in the right abdominal flank. Here the 4th- and 5th-stage larvae are found in association with hemorrhagic nodules 1 to several cm. in diameter. Some larvae may migrate between layers of the mesocolon to the wall of the cecum and colon where more hemorrhagic nodules may develop. This usually occurs 3-5 months after the original infection. Eventually young adults find their way to the lumen of the colon where they mature. Eggs are produced 300-320 days after infection. Larvae are sometimes found in the liver, lungs, testes, thoracic cavity, and beneath the pleura. Adults may also be found in hemorrhagic nodules or hematomas in the body cavity.

Transmission: Ingestion of 3rd-stage larvae with food and water. Most infective larvae die after a few months exposure on pasture, but some may survive over winter or as long as a year.

Signs and pathogenicity: Clinical signs appear slowly; feces become soft, diarrhea develops, and appetite diminishes. Animals become easily exhausted, and the hair coat becomes rough. Signs and lesions vary with parasite species and organs and tissues affected, e.g., *S. vulgaris* associated with thrombi and parasitic aneurysms. Thromboembolic colic, intermittent lameness in rear limbs, and a variety of other conditions may occur.

Diagnosis: By demonstration of eggs from feces, but larvae are required for specific identification. Rectal palpation for aneurysm involving the cranial mesenteric artery may be helpful.

Control: Avoid overstocking and overgrazing. Practice pasture rotation and mixed grazing. Proper stacking of manure to heat will destroy many infective forms. Phenothiazine as a therapeutic dose or added to feed at a low level is effective. Thiabendazole is highly effective against adult forms.

Selected references:

Drudge, J. H., E. T. Lyons, and J. Szanto. 1966. Pathogenesis of migrating stages of helminths, with special reference to *Strongylus vulgaris*. In *Biology of parasites*, ed. E. J. L. Soulsby, pp. 199-213. New York: Academic Press.

Farelly, B. T. 1954. The pathogenesis and significance of parasitic endarteritis and thrombosis in the ascending aorta of the horse. *Vet. Rec.* 66:53-61.

Ottaway, C. W., and M. L. Bingham. 1946. Further observations on the incidence of parasitic aneurysms in the horse. *Vet. Rec.* 58:155-59.

Ottaway, C. W., and M. L. Clarke. 1951. Further observations on the larval migration of *Strongylus vulgaris*. *Vet. Rec.* 63:444.

Poynter, D. 1960. The arterial lesions produced by *Strongylus vulgaris* and their relationship to the migratory route of the parasite in its host. *Res. Vet. Sci.* 1:205-17.

PARASITE: *Syngamus trachea* (gapeworm, gapes, Y-worm, forked worm)

Disease: Syngamiasis.
Host: Chicken, turkeys, guinea fowl, wild birds.
Habitat: Trachea.
Identification: When fresh, worms are usually bright red. The pattern of

males and females in permanent copulation resembles the letter Y. Males may be 6 mm. long, females about 20 mm. long. Eggs are 90 x 45 μ with an operculum at each pole.

Distribution and importance: Widely distributed; no longer very important to the poultry industry because current commercial management systems minimize infection. This helminth remains a problem in game birds and, occasionally, turkeys.

Life cycle: Birds may become infected directly by ingestion of embryonated eggs or infective larvae or indirectly by ingestion of earthworms containing free or encysted gapeworm larvae. It is suspected that other invertebrates may be paratenic hosts in which the larvae may remain viable for months or years. Gapeworm larvae may remain infective in the earthworm for $4^{1}/_{3}$ years. Passage through earthworms is thought to render larvae more highly infective enabling strains to transfer more readily from one bird species to another. After ingestion the infective larvae travel via the blood to the lungs and rupture the alveoli; then the young adults migrate via the air passages to the trachea. The prepatent period is 2-3 weeks, and the longevity of the adults is 4-8 months.

Transmission: By ingestion of the infective larva, an egg containing an infective larva, or the paratenic host carrying the infective larvae.

Signs and pathogenicity: Usually young birds are affected. They gasp for breath because of mechanical obstruction of the trachea by adult worms, mucus exudate, or nodule formation. Dyspnea and signs of asphyxia with convulsive head-shaking are common. Death may result from asphyxia or progressive emaciation and weakness.

Diagnosis: Observation of suffocation due to tracheal obstruction and demonstration of adult worms in the trachea of the live bird or at necropsy. Operculated eggs in the feces also may be identified.

Control: Avoid pens and yards with wet, organic soil suitable for earthworms. Place birds on fresh ground; do not mix chickens and turkeys. Wild birds, especially game birds, should be excluded from chicken runs insofar as this is possible. Barium antimony tartrate has proved a satisfactory inhalant for treatment. Thiabendazole at the rate of 0.5% in a medicated mash gives excellent results.

Selected references:

Harwood, P. D., and J. M. Schaffer. 1939. Barium antimonyl tartrate as a remedy for the removal of gapeworms from chickens. *Poultry Sc.* 18:63-65.

Wehr, E. E. 1941. Controlling gapeworm in poultry. *U.S.D.A. Leaflet #207.* Pp. 1-6.

Wehr, E. E., and J. C. Hwang. 1967. Anthelmintic activity of thiabendazole against the gapeworm (*Syngamus trachea*) in turkeys. *Avian Dis.* 11:44-48.

PARASITE: *Tetrameres americana, T. crami* (globular stomach worm)

Disease: Tetrameriasis.

Host: Poultry, ducks, and geese.

Habitat: Proventriculus.

Identification: The mature female worm is almost spherical or globular and blood-red. The slender male is cylindrical and is usually overlooked because it is small. Males are as long as 6 mm., and females are about 4 by 3 mm. The thick-shelled, elliptical egg, 45 by 25 μ, contains an embryo when passed in the feces.

Distribution and importance: Irregularly distributed throughout North America. Infections are usually light and of minor importance.

Life cycle: Eggs are eliminated in the feces and hatch after ingestion by an insect such as a grasshopper or cockroach (in the case of *T. americana*). Infection of birds follows ingestion of the infected arthropod. The prepatent period is almost 45 days. In the case of *T. crami*, the intermediate host is an amphipod.

Transmission: Ingestion of infected grasshopper, cockroach, or amphipod.

Signs and pathogenicity: Disease signs are seldom attributed to this parasite. Proventricular walls may thicken, and individuals may show signs of dullness and be emaciated. Subsequently they may die.

Diagnosis: Identification of nematodes on visual examination of proventricular glands.

Control: Raise birds on wire. Clean yards and runs of debris that provides cover for arthropods.

Selected references:

Cram, E. B. 1931. Developmental stages of some nematodes of the Spiruroidea parasitic in poultry and game birds. *U.S.D.A. Tech. Bul.* 227:1-27.

Swales, W. E. 1933. *Tetrameres crami* sp. nov., a nematode parasitizing the proventriculus of a domestic duck in Canada. *Can. J. Res.* 8:334-36.

PARASITE: *Thelazia californiensis* (eyeworm)

Disease: Thelaziasis.

Host: Dog, cat, sheep, deer, and rarely man.

Habitat: Tear-duct, conjunctival sac, and under the nictitating membrane.

Identification: Thin, filariform nematodes to 18 mm. long; a viviparous species.

Distribution and importance: Most prevalent on the west coast of North

America. Thelaziasis is easily treated, and although annoying to the infected animal, it is rarely of major importance.

Life cycle: The larvae, laid in the lachrymal secretions, are ingested by a muscid fly of such genera as *Musca* or *Fannia*. The larva develops in the thorax or abdomen of the fly and is infective in about 30 days. The larva then moves to the labium and migrates into the eye of a new host when the fly feeds. The prepatent period is 3-6 weeks.

Transmission: Infective larvae are transferred to a new host when the muscid feeds on the secretions of the eye.

Signs and pathogenicity: Usual signs are lachrymation, photophobia, and occasional conjunctivitis. Panophthalmia may result from heavy infections with bacterial involvement.

Diagnosis: Identification of embryonated eggs or larvae in lachrymal secretions or gross observation of the adults in the eye.

Control: Use of insecticides to reduce fly populations. Adult worms may be removed after applying a topical ophthalmic anesthetic. Irrigation of the conjunctival sac with a very mild solution of boric acid, mercuric chloride or iodine has been recommended.

Selected references:

Burnett, H. S., W. E. Parmelee, R. D. Lee, and E. D. Wagner. 1957. Observations on the life cycle of *Thelazia californiensis*, Price, 1930. *J. Parasitol.* 43:433.

Chitwood, M. B., and J. G. Stoffolano. 1971. First report of *Thelazia* sp. (Nematoda) in the face fly, *Musca autumnalis* in North America. *J. Parasitol.* 57:1363-64.

Parmalee, W. E., R. D. Lee, E. D. Wagner, and H. S. Burnett. 1956. A survey of *Thelazia californiensis*, a mammalian eye worm, with new locality records. *J. Am. Vet. Med. Assoc.* 129:325-27.

PARASITE: *Toxascaris leonina* (large roundworm)

Disease: Toxascariasis.

Host: Dog, cat, fox, and wild carnivores.

Habitat: Small intestine.

Identification: May be about 10 cm. long. The cervical alae give a lance-like appearance to the anterior end. The slightly ovoid egg has a smooth shell and is about 80 x 70 μ.

Distribution and importance: Widely distributed and commonly encountered throughout North America. It is not an important pathogen when limited to the intestine of older dogs, but it may contribute to the general unthriftiness and potbellied condition in pups if infection is severe.

Life cycle: Under optimal conditions, the egg becomes infective in 3-6 days and contains a 2nd-stage larva. After ingestion the egg hatches, and the larva enters the intestinal wall and remains there for about 2 weeks. Subsequently it molts and returns to the lumen to mature about 6 weeks after initial infection. There is no extensive larval migration like that of *Toxocara canis*; prenatal infection does not take place.

Transmission: Ingestion of infective egg or ingestion of a paratenic host such as a small rodent.

Signs and pathogenicity: An infected animal is usually unthrifty and may be potbellied; the coat is harsh and dull. Intermittent diarrhea and constipation may occur, and the animal may be slightly emaciated. Intestinal obstruction may occur in severe infections.

Diagnosis: Suggestive clinical signs may be confirmed by identifying eggs from the feces or adult worms in the droppings or vomitus of the host.

Control: General sanitation, regular treatment of young dogs, and eradication of rodent paratenic hosts.

Selected references:

Sprent, J. F. A. 1959. The life history and development of *Toxascaris leonina* in dog and cat. *Parasitology* 49:330-71.

Sprent, J. F. A., and M. G. Barrett. 1964. Large roundworms of dogs and cats: differentiation of *Toxocara canis* and *Toxascaris leonina*. *Aust. Vet. Jour.* 40:166-71.

PARASITE: *Toxocara canis*, *T. cati* (syn. *mystax*) (large roundworm of dog and cat)

Disease: Toxocariasis.

Host: *T. canis:* dog, fox. *T. cati:* cat.

Habitat: Small intestine; somatic tissues (*T. canis* only).

Identification: *T. canis:* May be 18 cm. long; the subglobular egg, about 85 μ in diameter, is finely pitted. The head end bears large, lanceolate, cervical alae. *T. cati:* May be 10 cm. long; egg is 65 x 75 μ. The cervical alae are broad, striated, and arrowhead-shaped.

Distribution and importance: Widely distributed throughout North America; of considerable economic importance to dog owners and kennels raising many dogs.

Life cycle: *T. canis:* This life cycle includes both hepatic-tracheal and somatic modes of migration. After passage in the feces, the eggs become infective in 10-15 days depending on temperature and humidity. Infective eggs hatch on ingestion, and the 2nd-stage larva penetrates the intestinal mucosa. Depending on age and sex of the host, the larva may then follow the tracheal route of migration or become established in the somatic tissues of the adult host. The latter is more common in the female dog. The tracheal migration occurs routinely in young dogs less than 5-6 weeks of age. In older dogs fewer larvae reach the trachea; the majority appear to enter the systemic circulation via the lungs and then migrate to the somatic tissues and organs. In dogs older than 6 months, the migration is almost entirely somatic, and few adult worms are found in the small intestine. When a bitch becomes pregnant, the larvae find their way across the placental barrier to the lungs of the fetus. It seems reasonable to assume that the mechanism that induces mobilization of the larvae is hormonal. Thus the bitch may have repeated infected litters even though she was free of adult *Toxocara* before her 1st pregnancy. If *Toxocara* eggs are ingested, the prepatent period is 4-5 weeks. If infection is prenatal, eggs are first passed about 4 weeks after birth. In addition this parasite may be acquired through a paratenic host. Thus the life cycle may include prey such as small mammals and birds serving as transport hosts.

T. cati: The life cycle of this parasite differs radically from that of *T. canis* because prenatal infection does not occur. The infection is acquired by ingesting the egg containing a 2nd-stage larva. In the stomach the larva emerges, penetrates the mucosa, and follows the hepatic-tracheal migratory route. The final molt to the adult occurs in the lumen of the small intestine. Transport hosts are varied and may be earthworms, beetles, and small mammals, especially mice. The prepatent period is about 55 days.

Transmission: *T. canis:* Through ingestion of infective eggs or an infected transport host. Transplacental and transmammary routes are also important. *T. cati:* Through ingestion of infective eggs or by ingestion of an infected transport host, especially a mouse. Transmammary infection may also occur.

Signs and pathogenicity: In the young dog, the usual signs are unthriftiness, potbelly with tucked-up abdomen, a dull harsh coat, emaciation, and, occasionally, intestinal obstruction. In initial heavy infections, submucosal hemorrhage and enteritis may occur. During larval migration, lobular pneumonia may cause death in heavily, prenatally infected pups. Adult worms in the digestive tract may be associated with a potbellied condition and some diarrhea; the pup does not do well. Pups may die 2-3 weeks after birth. Nervous signs have been attributed to toxocariasis, but this suggestion requires cautious interpretation. At present *Toxocara canis* is implicated as the prime etiologic agent responsible for the visceral type of larva migrans in children (4 years or younger).

Diagnosis: The characteristic globular eggs with thick, pitted shells are readily recognized. Whole worms in vomitus or feces may be identified.

Control: Adult worms may be satisfactorily removed with piperazine and organic phosphorus compounds. The maternal reservoirs of infection present the greatest problem in control until we have an anthelmintic that will kill larva in situ in the somatic tissues. For complete control an appropriate program of medication and strict sanitation must be planned by the owner and the veterinarian. Thus bitches carrying somatic infections may be gradually cleared of somatic larvae after several pregnancies. Because rodents, other small mammals, and birds may be transport hosts for this parasite, their control and elimination must be considered a routine management procedure.

Selected references:
> Griesemer, R. A., and J. P. Gibson. 1963. The establishment of an ascarid-free beagle dog colony. *J. Am. Vet. Med. Assoc.* 143:965-67.
> Sprent, J. F. A. 1956. Life history and development of *Toxocara cati. Parasitology* 46:54-78.
> ———. 1958. Observations on the development of *Toxocara canis* in the dog. *Parasitology* 48:184-209.
> Swerczek, T. W., S. W. Nielsen, and C. F. Helmboldt. 1971. Transmammary passage of *Toxocara cati* in the cat. *Am. J. Vet. Res.* 32:89-92.
> Yutuc, L. M. 1949. Prenatal infection of dogs with ascarids, *Toxocara canis*, and hookworms, *Ancylostoma caninum. J. Parasitol.* 35:358-60.

PARASITE: *Trichinella spiralis* (trichina worm)

Disease: Trichinelliasis, trichinosis.

Host: Man, pig, rat, and most other flesh-eating mammals; birds experimentally. The definitive host and intermediate host may be the same animal in this life cycle.

Habitat: Small intestine of definitive host, musculature of intermediate host.

Identification: Body fine and slender. The female may be 4 mm. long; the male is smaller. The posterior end of the male bears lateral flaps on either side of the cloacal opening. The egg is 40 x 30 μ and contains a fully developed embryo when in the uterus of the female.

Distribution: Widely distributed throughout North America. In swine the prevalence is about 0.125% in farm-raised swine and 0.5% in garbage-fed hogs. The infection in man is about 4.0%.

Life cycle: On ingestion of infected meat the cyst wall is dissolved by gastric juice, and the larva is liberated. It develops rapidly and matures in 2-3 days. The male dies a few days after copulation. The female penetrates deeply the mucosa of the small intestine and reaches the lymph spaces of the villi. It lives for about 6 weeks and produces living larvae in vast numbers during the first 2 weeks. The larva enters the lymph channels and moves to the thoracic duct. From the 8th to the 25th day after infection, it is carried throughout the body by the peripheral circulation. The larva then leaves the capillaries and penetrates the sarcolemma of the striated muscle fibers, rich in blood supply. The larva grows rapidly and in 30 days is about 1 mm. long. The cyst wall develops around the larva in about 3 months, and the cyst is then 0.4-0.6 mm. by 0.25 mm. The cyst usually calcifies in 6-8 months, but the larva may live for many years (to 11 years in the hog). Mammals may serve as both definitive and intermediate hosts.

Transmission: Ingestion of infected muscle; possibly ingestion of infected feces.

Signs and pathogenicity: Clinical signs are seldom observed in domestic or wild animals. In man clinical signs are highly variable. During the intestinal stage and the period of invasion, the clinical signs may be nonspecific gastroenteritis, i.e., nausea, vomiting, watery diarrhea, malaise, and fever. During the period of larval migration there may be a severe myositis, muscle pain, and an eosinophilia (15-50% or higher). Death most frequently occurs during the 4th-6th week. In the period of encystment and repair, the signs seen during larval migration may be exaggerated, and death may result from exhaustion, pneumonia, or cardiac failure.

Diagnosis: In domestic animals, a diagnosis is seldom made. An absolute diagnosis is made by demonstration of encysted larvae in skeletal muscle. This may be accomplished by use of a compressorium or a muscle-digestion procedure. Other laboratory diagnostic aids and procedures are blood examination for an eosinophilia, demonstration of adults in feces, muscle biopsy, and the precipitin or intracutaneous test.

Control: Measures are designed to prevent spread among pigs, reveal presence of trichinae in hog carcasses, and render infective pork safe. These goals are accomplished by cooking garbage fed to hogs, examining each pig slaughtered, and chemically or physically treating pork to be consumed raw or semi-cooked. Larvae are killed at 55°C. For safety when cooking pork the deepest portion of the meat should reach 58.3°C. If relying on cold to kill larvae, small pieces of meat (not thicker than 6 in.) should be stored at −15°C. for not fewer than 20 days. Pork should be cooked until it loses its pink color. To remove *T. spiralis* from the definitive host, thiabendazole is the drug of choice, though its undesirable side effects must be considered.

Selected references:

Gould, S. E. 1970. *Trichinosis in man and animals*. Springfield, Ill.: Thomas.

Leighty, J. C. 1974. The role of meat inspection in preventing *Trichinosis* in man. *J. Am. Vet. Med. Assoc.* 165:994-95.

Zimmerman, W. J. 1971. The trichiniasis problem: facts, fallacies and future. *Iowa State Univ. Vet.* 33:93-97.

Zimmerman, W. J., and J. H. Steele. 1973. Trichinosis in the U.S. population, 1966-70. *Health Services Reports. U.S. Dept. H. E. W.* 88:606-23.

PARASITE: *Trichostrongylus axei* (stomach hair worm)

Disease: Trichostrongylosis.

Host: Equine species, also cattle and sheep.

Habitat: Lumen of gastric glands, occasionally duodenum.

Identification: Slender, reddish-brown worms, to 5.5 mm. long. Eggs are 85 x ?5 μ.

Distribution and importance: Generally throughout North America but probably seldom observed. Its economic importance is questionable. No fatal infections of this parasite have been reported. The horse may acquire infection as a result of mixed grazing with cattle and sheep.

Life cycle: Direct. The prepatent period is 20-25 days. Eggs are passed in the host's feces, and infective larvae develop in 4-6 days under optimal environmental conditions. Little development occurs below $9°C$.

Transmission: Ingestion of infective larvae.

Signs and pathogenicity: Heavy infections may cause a mild catarrhal gastritis. Isolated raised areas of the glandular mucosa may devleop, especially in the fundic area. Such circumscribed areas may be half to several centimeters in diameter and have a depressed craterlike center. Changes in the mucosa take place very slowly, and most infections are chronic and mild in nature.

Diagnosis: Because all strongylate eggs are similar, it is difficult to identify eggs of this species. At necropsy, skin scrapings of the gastric mucosa should be made to demonstrate adult worms.

Control: Grazing management. Avoid grazing horses with ruminants unless pastures have lain idle. Weathering and desiccation kill larvae. Thiabendazole is probably the drug of choice if control is indicated.

Selected references:

Douvres, F. W. 1957. The morphogenesis of the parasitic stages of *Trichostrongylus axei* and *Trichostrongylus colubriformis* nematode parasites of cattle. *Proc. Helm. Soc. Wash.* 24:4-14.

Roth, H., and N. O. Christensen. 1942. On parasitic gastritis in the horse due to *Trichostrongylus axei. Skand. Vet. Tidskr.* 32:488-514.

PARASITE: *Trichostrongylus colubriformis, T. vitrinus, T. capricola, T. facultatus, T. rugatus, T. longispicularis,* (hair worm, bankrupt worm, black scours worm)

Disease: Trichostrongylosis.

Host: Ruminants, but has occasionally been reported from man, pig, and horse.

Habitat: Throughout small intestine. *T. colubriformis* is sometimes in the abomasum.

Identification: Threadlike, pale, reddish worms. The thin-shelled egg is oval and segmenting when laid. It is 80-90 by 40-45 μ. The cuticle has annular striations; longitudinal ridges are not present. The adult is 5-8 mm. long.

Distribution and importance: Generally North America. Owing to their small size adults are frequently overlooked. This is an important group of nematodes.

Life cycle: The typical thin-shelled, strongylelike eggs develop to infective 3rd-stage larvae in 1-7 days. Below 9°C. little or no development occurs. Migration of larvae on grass is influenced by light intensity. High temperature and dryness are destructive to larvae, and it is unlikely that many larvae survive more than 4-6 months on pasture. Some overwintering on pasture may occur.

Transmission: Ingestion of infective larvae with food or water.

Signs and pathogenicity: Mixed infections are usually seen in ovine and bovine trichostrongylidosis. Disease may be acute; animals may be very weak and die. In chronic cases the skin becomes dry, constipation and diarrhea alternate, and dark, diarrheic feces are common; hence the name "black scours worm." Intestinal forms penetrate mucosae and produce irregular circumscribed thickenings.

Diagnosis: Identification of worms at necropsy is the most certain method of diagnosis. Fecal examinations and egg counts are of limited value.

Control: Grazing management is important in control; however, anthelmintic medication is usually necessary. Anthelmintics of great efficacy currently available are thiabendazole, tetramisole, ruelene, haloxon, and others. Regular treatment, good feed, and a planned management program should be routinely followed.

Selected references:

Douvres, F. W. 1957. The morphogenesis of the parasitic stages of *Trichostrongylus axei* and *Trichostrongylus colubriformis*, nematode parasites of cattle. *Proc. Helm. Soc. Wash.* 24:4-14.

Gibson, T. E. 1954. Studies on trichostrongylosis. 1. Pathogenesis of *T. axei* in sheep maintained on a low plane of nutrition. *Jour. Comp. Path. and Thera.* 64:127-40.

Keith, R. K. 1953. The differentiation of the infective larvae of some common nematode parasites of cattle. *Aust. J. Zool.* 1:223-35.

PARASITE: *Trichuris ovis* (whipworm)

Disease: Trichuriasis.

Host: Sheep, goat, and cattle.

Habitat: Cecum and occasionally colon.

Identification: May be about 8 cm. long. The long filamentous anterior end is almost twice as long as the thicker posterior end. The worm is whitish. The whiplike shape and habitat make identification easy. The egg is typical of the genus because it is lemon-shaped, yellow to brown, and has a transparent polar plug at each end. The egg is about 80 x 40 μ including the plugs.

Distribution and importance: Generally throughout North America.

Life cycle: Under favorable conditions, eggs may reach the infective stage in about 3 weeks. Development may be prolonged at low temperatures. Infective eggs may remain viable for several years. On ingestion the eggs hatch, and the larvae migrate to the cecum to mature in 1-3 months.

Transmission: Infection is acquired by ingestion of the infective egg.

Signs and pathogenicity: No pathogenic significance has ever been claimed for *T. ovis* in cattle, and it is seldom recognized as a serious pathogen of sheep. In lambs heavy infections have been associated with diarrhea and occasional flecks of blood in the feces.

Diagnosis: Identification of eggs in feces.

Control: Accomplished by a general parasite-control program for the flock or herd.

Selected references:

Burrows, R. B., and W. G. Lillis. 1964. The whipworm as a bloodsucker. *J. Parasitol.* 50:675-80.

Farleigh, E. A. 1966. Observations on the pathogenic effects of *Trichuris ovis* in sheep under drought conditions. *Aust. Vet. J.* 42:462-63.

PARASITE: *Trichuris suis* (whipworm)

Disease: Trichuriasis.

Host: Pig.

Habitat: Cecum, colon.

Identification: Anterior part of the body long and slender; posterior part much thicker. The adult may be 5 cm. long. The yellow to brown egg, about 55 x 25 μ, has transparent plugs at each pole.

Distribution and importance: Throughout North America in pig-raising areas.

Life cycle: Eggs become infective in about 3 weeks at suitable temperatures. Development may be delayed at temperatures below 20°C. Once infective, eggs may remain viable for several years. The prepatent period is about 6 weeks but may be much longer.

Transmission: Ingestion of infective eggs.

Signs and pathogenicity: Opinions vary regarding the pathogenicity of this nematode. There is little doubt that an acute or chronic cecitis or colitis may result from heavy infections. In animals experimentally infected, hemorrhagic necrosis and edema of the cecal mucosa have been observed. A watery hemorrhagic diarrhea and growth retardation have been reported in acute infections. Clinical signs in young pigs are anorexia, diarrhea, incoordination, and emaciation; some deaths may occur after weaning.

Diagnosis: Demonstration of characteristic lemon-shaped eggs in the feces and identification of worms on necropsy.

Control: Because the eggs may remain viable on soil for 6 years, *T. suis* is difficult to control. Hogs may have to be moved to clean pasture or range so that the contaminated pasture can be left fallow and then cultivated until safe for hogs. Hygromycin in feed and trichlorfon intramuscularly are claimed to be effective treatments. Dichlorvos in uncoated resin pellets is also claimed effective. Eggs are susceptible to desiccation. Use of the McClean County Swine Sanitation System should help in control of this parasite.

Selected references:

Batte, E. G., and D. J. Moncol. 1972. Whipworms and dysentery in feeder pigs. *J. Am. Vet. Med. Assoc.* 161:1226-28.

Powers, K. G., A. C. Todd, and S. H. McNutt. 1960. Experimental infections of swine with *Trichuris suis*. *Am. J. Vet. Res.* 21:262-68.

Schoneweis, D. A., and W. R. Rapp. 1970. *Trichuris suis* infection in young pigs. *Vet. Med. Sm. Anim. Clin.* 65:63-66.

PARASITE: *Trichuris vulpis* (whipworm)

Disease: Trichuriasis.

Host: Dog, fox.

Habitat: Cecum and large intestine.

Identification: Whiplike shape of the worm makes identification simple. It may be 75 mm. long, of which three-quarters is the anterior, slender portion of the worm. The egg, typical of the genus, is lemon-shaped with a polar plug at each end. The egg is about 75 x 40 μ.

Distribution and importance: Generally distributed throughout North America. Their significance seems to depend on the number present.

Life cycle: Under favorable conditions the egg becomes infective in about 3 weeks and may remain viable for several years. The egg is highly resistant to freezing but susceptible to desiccation. After ingestion the infective egg hatches, and the larva reaches the cecum and matures in 1-3 months.

Transmission: By ingestion of infective eggs with food and water.

Signs and pathogenicity: Opinions vary concerning the pathogenicity of the nematode. In heavy infections acute and chronic typhlitis have been observed. Such signs as unthriftiness, loss of weight, diarrhea, and dysentery have been associated with large numbers of this parasite. *T. vulpis* feeds on blood.

Diagnosis: Demonstration of the characteristic lemon-shaped egg in the feces. The egg must be differentiated from that of *Capillaria* sp. which is similar.

Control: Kennels, runs, and exercise pens should be cleaned thoroughly and allowed to dry in direct sunlight and should have good drainage. Several anthelmintics such as whipcide, glycobiarsol, and dichlorvos are claimed to be highly effective.

Selected references:

Miller, M. J. 1939. *Trichocephalus* and trichocephaliasis. *Can. J. Comp. Med.* 3:282-87.

Rubin, R. 1954. Studies on the common whipworm of the dog, *Trichuris vulpis*. *Cornell Vet.* 44:36-49.

PARASITE: *Triodontophorus* (6 spp.), *Craterostomum* (1 sp.), *Oesophagodontus* (1 sp.), *Gyalocephalus* (1 sp.), *Trichonema* (34 spp.) (small strongyles, small redworms, or blood worms)

Disease: Strongylidosis.

Host: Equine species.

Habitat: Mostly large intestine, cecum.

Identification: These small strongyles do not migrate. *Triodontophorus* and *Oesophagodontus* may be 22 mm. long; members of the other 3 genera are 6-12 mm. long. The species are identified on the basis of presence of external and internal leaf crowns and of teeth projecting into the buccal capsule.

Distribution and importance: Prevalent wherever horses are found. Larval stages cause considerable economic loss and may produce severe disease if present in large numbers.

Life cycle: After ingestion infective larvae exsheath and enter the intestinal mucosa where they may remain for 2-3 months. Fourth-stage larvae return to the lumen of the large intestine, molt, and mature. Infective larvae embedded in the mucosa appear to be inhibited in their development by the presence of adult worms in the lumen of the intestine. Gibson (1957) demonstrated that using anthelmintics to remove adult worms will permit development of inhibited larvae to maturity.

Transmission: Ingestion of infective larvae with food or water.

Signs and pathogenicity: Catarrhal enteritis has been attributed to the presence of large numbers of adult small strongyles. The larval form is reputed to ingest blood and has been associated with cases of winter anemia in horses. The larvae cause formation of nodules varying from a minute speck to a body about 6 mm. in diameter. Within each nodule may usually be found a coiled, black or reddish larva. If the larva fails to escape from the nodule, permanent encapsulation may take place.

Diagnosis: Specific diagnosis can only be made with the aid of larval cultures and differential morphological studies.

Control: Adult stock should be treated at least every 3 months during the pasture season. Currently a wide selection of highly effective anthelmintics is available. Mixed grazing with sheep or cattle is a better means of reducing the helminth pasture burden than is simply allowing the pasture to rest. In a confined area such as a box stall or a small paddock or pasture, the manure should be removed each day. This will greatly reduce the contamination of the pasture. Piperazine has been shown to be highly effective against *Trichonema* sp. Thiabendazole is also effective against this group and is claimed to be effective against larval forms. To control these helminths a program of routine medication should be followed by the owner. Clean water supplies, raised hay racks and feed bunks, and collection and composting of horse manure should be routine procedures in any parasite-control program.

Selected references:

Downing, W., P. A. Kingsbury, and J. E. N. Sloan. 1955. Critical tests with piperazine adipate in horses. *Vet. Rec.* 67:641-44.

Drudge, J. H., S. E. Leland, Z. N. Wyant, G. W. Elam, C. E. Smith and E. Dale. 1957. Critical tests with piperazine-carbon disulfide complex (Parvex) against parasites of the horse. *Am. J. Vet. Res.* 18:792-97.

Gibson, T. E. 1957. Critical tests of piperazine adipate as an equine anthelmintic. *Br. Vet. J.* 113:90-92.

PARASITE: *Uncinaria stenocephala* (northern dog hookworm, northern hookworm)

Disease: Uncinariasis.

Host: Dog, cat.

Habitat: Small intestine, frequently in posterior third.

Identification: A small nematode which may be about 12.0 mm. long. The buccal capsule is characterized by a pair of broad cutting plates instead of teeth on the ventral border. Dorsal teeth are absent. The egg is about 70 x 45 μ.

Distribution and importance: This hookworm has a northerly distribution and thus is found most frequently in the colder regions of North America.

Life cycle: Similar to that of *A. caninum*. The larva is infective in about 4 days. If ingested, the larva develops directly without any systemic migration. The prepatent period is about 15 days. This species appears to be better adapted to developing at low temperatures than other members of the Anycylostomidae.

Transmission: Usually by ingestion of infective larvae. Percutaneous infection does not seem to be very successful.

Signs and pathogenicity: This helminth is slightly pathogenic and seldom seems associated with clinical disease in dogs in northern regions.

Diagnosis: Demonstration of eggs in feces.

Control: Similar to that appropriate for *Ancylostoma caninum*.

Selected references:

Gibbs, H. C. 1961. Studies on the life cycle and developmental morphology of *Dochmoides stenocephala*. *Can. J. Zool.* 39:325-48.

B. Cestodes

For *Coenurus* sp. and *Cysticercus* sp. life cycles see *Taenia*.

PARASITE: *Anoplocephala magna, A. perfoliata, Paranoplocephala mamillana* (tapeworm)

Disease: Anoplocephaliasis.

Host: Horses, donkeys.

Habitat: *A. magna*: Small intestine, occasionally stomach. *A. perfoliata*: Small and large intestine and cecum. It frequently occurs in colonies around the ileocecal valve. *P. mamillana*: Small intestine, occasionally stomach.

Identification: *A. magna*: To 80 cm. long; scolex pronounced. Egg is 50-60 μ. *A. perfoliata*: To 8 cm. long; small head with lappets posterior to each sucker. Egg is 65-80 μ. *P. mamillana*: To 4 cm. long; suckers slitlike. Egg is 50 μ.

Distribution and importance: *A. magna*: Cosmopolitan; not generally considered very important. *A perfoliata*: Heavy infections may significantly interfere with function of the ileocecal valve. *P. mamillana*: Seldom of much importance.

Life cycle: *A. magna*: Cysticercoids are produced in oribatid mites, namely, *Scheloribates laevigatus* and *S. latipes*. *A. perfoliata*: Larval development occurs in the following mites: *Scheloribates laevigatus, S. latipes, Galumna obvious, G. nervosus, Achiperia* spp., and *Seratozetes* spp. *P. mamillana*: Intermediate hosts are the mites *Galumna obvious* and *Allogalumna longipluma*. Infected mites are ingested on herbage, and adult tapeworms are found in the intestine in 4-6 weeks. Cysticercoids in mites become infective in 2-4 months.

Transmission: Ingestion of oribatid mite infected with appropriate cysticercoid.

Signs and pathogenicity: Mild infections of these species are not associated with clinical signs. Heavy infections of *A. perfoliata* may be associated with ulcerous depressions at the point of attachment by the tapeworm. Function of the ileocecal valve may be impaired, thus recurrent attacks of colic may occur. It is claimed that *A. magna* may initiate a catarrhal and sometimes hemorrhagic inflammation of the intestines.

Diagnosis: Presence in feces of tapeworm segments or eggs with characteristic pyriform apparatus.

Control: Widespread occurrence of mites on pasture makes prevention very difficult. Oil of chenopodium, malefern, and oil of turpentine have been used to remove horse tapeworms. Bithionol has been reported to be effective but is not available at present.

Selected references:

Fukui, M., C. Kaneko, and A. Ogawa. 1960. Studies on equine tapeworms and their intermediate hosts. II. Studies on removal effects of bithionol, bithionol acetate, and dichlorophen for equine tapeworm, *Anoplocephala perfoliata*. *Jap. J. Parasitol.* 9:217-23.

PARASITE: *Coenurus cerebralis* (Adult is *Taenia multiceps*)

Disease: Coenurosis cerebralis, gid, sturdy.

Host: Intermediate hosts are sheep, cattle, goats, and horses; definitive hosts are dogs, coyotes, and foxes.

Habitat: Small intestine for the adult. Brain and spinal cord for larvae in the ovine intermediate host.

Identification: Adult to 100 cm. long; small scolex with 22-32 hooks. The uterus has 9-26 lateral branches on both sides of the main stem; eggs are 29-37 μ diameter. The full-grown coenurus is about 5 cm. in diameter.

Distribution and importance: Distribution uncertain in the U.S.; claimed to have been reported from sheep in Montana. It is of little economic significance in the U.S.

Life cycle: Tapeworm segments are passed in the dog's feces, and eggs are ingested by sheep on pasture or in pens and yards. Eggs hatch in the sheep's intestine. The onchosphere passes through the intestinal wall to the bloodstream and then is carried throughout the body. If it reaches the C.N.S. it develops, otherwise it dies. The coernurus (bladderworm) becomes fully developed after 7-8 months in the brain. A carnivore then ingests the bladderworm, and the adult develops in 3-4 weeks. The coenurus has a delicate translucent wall, and several hundred scolexlike structures may be seen on the inner germinal wall of the cyst.

Transmission: By ingestion of the bladderworm (coenurus).

Signs and pathogenicity: The signs seen in the sheep depend upon the site of the coenurus in the central nervous system. Locomotor disturbance is common, and the disease is known as "sturdy" or "gid". The animal may hold its head to one side, circle, or lose its balance. Blindness and convulsions may be seen. Clinical signs are varied and depend upon the location of the bladderworm. Signs usually appear 2-7 months after initial infection.

Diagnosis: By identification of the adult from a carnivore or of the coenurus from the intermediate host.

Control: Destroy bladderworms in carcasses and prevent their ingestion by the definitive host. Treat sheep dogs regularly for tapeworms.

Selected references:

Becklund, W. W. 1970. Current knowledge of the gid bladder worm, *Coenurus cerebralis* (=*Taenia multiceps*), in North American domestic sheep, *Ovis aries*. *Proc. Helminthol. Soc. Wash.* 37:200-03.

Esch, G. W., and J. T. Self. 1965. A critical study of the taxonomy of *Taenia pisiformis* Block, 1780; *Multiceps multiceps* Leske, 1780; and *Hydatigena taeniaformis*. *J. Parasitol.* 51:932-37.

PARASITE: *Coenurus serialis* (bladderworm), (Adult is *Taenia serialis*)

Disease: Coenurosis.

Host: Rabbit, hare, horse, squirrel.

Habitat: Adult in intestine of carnivore; larval stage in intermuscular connective tissue of hare, rabbit, and squirrel.

Identification: Adult may be 70 cm. long. The elliptical egg is 30 x 35 μ. The full-grown bladderworm is about 4 cm. long; its numerous solices are arranged in lines.

Distribution and importance: Throughout North America; of minor economic importance.

Life cycle: Larval stage, *C. serialis*, develops in intermuscular connective tissue of hare, squirrel, and rabbit. The dog acquires the adult worm by ingesting raw flesh of an infected rodent or lagomorph. Each scolex ingested develops into a tapeworm.

Transmission: Ingestion of a coenurus by eating raw flesh of an infected rodent or lagomorph.

Signs and pathogenicity: Not particularly pathogenic, but may possibly interfere with muscle function.

Diagnosis: Identification of adult worm from carnivore or coenurus from musculature of intermediate host.

Control: Do not feed raw rabbit to dogs; cook or freeze rabbits before feeding. Treat dogs with a taeniacide.

PARASITE: *Cysticercus bovis* (Adult is *Taenia saginata*) (beef tapeworm of man, unarmed tapeworm)

Disease: Bovine cysticercosis, beef measles (taeniasis in man).

Host: *C. bovis:* cattle. *T. saginata:* man.

Habitat: Intermuscular connective tissue, particularly of the masseter, heart, diaphragm, and tongue. In severe infections it may be found in other organs and tissues such as the liver, lungs, kidney, and abdominal fat.

Identification: Scolex without rostellum or hooks. The strobila is 4-10 meters long. Gravid segments have 15-35 lateral branches on both sides of the uterine stem. The egg is 40 x 25 μ. The oval cysticercus is translucent and grey-white with an invaginated scolex appearing as a dense white blob about 6-10 mm.

Distribution and importance: Of minor importance as a pathogen of animals including humans in North America. Economic importance is the cost of the inspection program to detect cysticerci in cattle. Heavily infected carcasses are condemned.

Life cycle: Gravid segments are passed in the feces. These are actively motile for a period, and eggs are shed as the segments move around and contract on drying. The egg is ingested by the bovine intermediate host, and the hexacanth embryo is liberated in the stomach. The freed onchosphere penetrates the intestinal mucosa, reaches the bloodstream, and may be carried to almost any organ or tissue. Owing to selective tissue requirements, it will develop only if it reaches a preferred tissue. The larva is fully infective in 2-3 months. The definitive host is infected by ingesting muscle containing a viable cysticercus. Cysticerci begin to degenerate 4-6 months after infection, and after 9 months a number may be dead depending on extent of infection and age of the intermediate host. In light infections the cysticerci may remain viable for a couple of years or longer. Most onchospheres die in less than 3 weeks on hay, but they will survive about 5 months on grass exposed to air. They will live 33 days in water and 71 days in liquid manure.

Transmission: By ingestion of viable cysticerci in bovine muscle; ingestion of rare beef by man. Cattle acquire the infection by ingesting grass, forage crops, or silage contaminated with tapeworm eggs released from gravid segments passed in the feces of man. Birds may also be mechanical vectors, carrying eggs on their feet or in their digestive tracts.

Signs and pathogenicity: Few clinical signs accompany an infection of man with the adult form. Diarrhea and hunger are most frequently noted. Under ordinary conditions cysticerci in cattle are not associated with clinical disease. Experimentally, massive infections in calves may cause such signs as anorexia, salivation, muscle stiffness, and degenerative myocarditis.

Diagnosis: Finding cysticerci with unarmed scolices in the muscle of the bovine carcass. The muscles commonly invaded are the masseter, tongue, heart, and diaphragm. In man, identification of gravid segments from the stool.

Control: Avoid using human manure or sewage for fertilization of cattle pastures. Cook meat for human consumption to at least 57°C. Meat should be uniformly grey in color. Freeze meat at −8 to −10°C. for 10 days or long enough to freeze the fluid within the cysticerci, rendering them noninfective. Adults in man may be removed with Yomesan.

Selected references:

Jepsen, A., and H. Roth. 1949. Epizootiology of *Cysticercus bovis*—Resistance of the eggs of *Taenia saginata*. *Proc. 14th Intl. Vet. Congress*, London. 2:43-50.

Pawlowski, Z., and M. G. Schultz. 1972. Taeniasis and cysticercosis (*Taenia saginata*). *Adv. Parasitol.* ed. B. Dawes. 10:269-304.

Urquart, G. M. 1961. Epizootiological and experimental studies on bovine cysticercosis in East Africa. *Jour. Parasitol.* 47:857-69.

Viljoen, N. F. 1937. Cysticercosis in swine and bovines, with special reference to South African conditions. *Onderstepoort J. Vet. Sc. An. Ind.* 9:337-570.

PARASITE: *Cysticercus cellulosae* (Adult is *Taenia solium*) (armed tapeworm, pork bladderworm)

Disease: Porcine cysticercosis, pork measles.

Host: Man is the definitive host and may be an intermediate host on occasion. The pig is the intermediate host. Many other mammals have been implicated as intermediate hosts, but the identifications may have been erroneous. Dog and sheep may harbor the cysticerci.

Habitat: Cysticerci usually are found in striated muscle, particularly the heart, tongue, and muscles of the thigh and neck, but may develop in other tissues and organs such as lung, liver, kidney, and brain. Adults are found in the small intestine of man. Ingestion of tapeworm eggs in contaminated food, from contaminated fingers, or by reverse peristalsis may cause human cysticercosis. Then cysticerci may be found in almost any human tissue, though subcutaneous tissues, eye, and brain are commonly invaded.

Identification: Adult may be 10 meters long. The rostellum bears 22-32 hooks in 2 rows. The uterus in the gravid segment has 7-12 lateral branches on both sides of the main stem. The cysticercus has an armed scolex.

Distribution and importance: Not frequently seen in the U.S.; rare in countries with adequate meat inspection. It is most common where hogs have access to feed or soil contaminated with human feces containing infective eggs. It is common in some regions of South America.

Life cycle: Eggs are ingested by the pig, and a hexacanth embryo is liberated in the intestine. The onchosphere enters the submucosal blood vessels and travels to the liver and subsequently throughout the body. It is principally found in striated muscle but is also found in other tissues and organs. In the pig, the cysticercus requires about 10 weeks for complete growth to about 10 x 20 mm. The cysts may remain viable for 2 years. Man is the only known definitive host for *T. solium*. Infection is acquired by ingestion of viable cysticerci in raw or inadequately cooked pork. In the stomach the pork flesh is digested, the head evaginates, and the larva attaches to the wall of the small intestine. It matures in 5-12 weeks. The adult worm may live 10 years.

Transmission: To man by ingesting raw pork containing viable cysticerci. To swine by ingesting food contaminated with human feces containing eggs.

Signs and pathogenicity: The adult tapeworm in man causes only a slight intestinal inflammation from the mechanical irritation of the mucosa by the strobila and the scolex. There is little reaction in man to the live cysticercus, but the dead cysticercus serves as a foreign body irritant. As a rule, the pig shows no clinical signs; however, paralysis of the tongue and convulsions have been attributed to this helminth.

Diagnosis: Detection on gross examination in meat inspection. Microscopic examination of cysticerci to identify the armed scolex is required for differential diagnosis. Serological tests have not proved satisfactory.

Control: Accomplished by education, sanitation, and an adequate meat inspection service. Hogs must not have access to human feces. Cysticerci are killed by freezing pork at $-10°C$. for 4 days or heating to $50°C$. Pickling cannot be relied upon to kill the cysticerci. Removal of adult worms is most readily accomplished with Yomesan. Dichlorophen is also effective. No anthelmintic treatment is available to destroy cysticerci in the tissues.

Selected references:

Viljoen, N. F. 1937. Cysticercosis in swine and bovines with special reference to South African conditions. *Onderstepoort J. Vet. Sc. An. Ind.* 9:337-570.

PARASITE: *Cysticercus ovis* (Adult is *Taenia ovis*)

Disease: Ovine cysticercosis, sheep measles.

Host: The intermediate host is the sheep; the definitive host is the dog or fox.

Habitat: Heart, diaphragm, and other skeletal muscle; under the epicardium and pleura of diaphragm as well.

Identification: Small oval cyst about 5 x 9.0 mm., a pea-sized vesicle.

Distribution and importance: Very low incidence in western North America; could be mistaken for *Cysticercus cellulosae*.

Life cycle: Similar to that of *C. cellulosae* (*Taenia solium*).

Transmission: Sheep ingest eggs from feces of a carnivore. The carnivore is infected by ingestion of cysticerci in sheep muscle.

Signs and pathogenicity: Not of major significance.

Selected references:

Gemmell, M. A. 1970. Hydatidosis and cysticercosis. 2. Distribution of *Cysticercus ovis* in sheep. *Austral. Vet. J.* 46:22-24.

PARASITE: *Cysticercus tenuicollis* (Adult is *Taenia hydatigena*) (thin-necked bladderworm)

Disease: Cysticercosis.

Host: Definitive hosts are carnivores; intermediate hosts may be sheep, goats, cattle, pigs, squirrels, hamsters, and wild ruminants.

Habitat: Usually found in the peritoneal cavity, on the mesentery, omentum, and other peritoneal surfaces.

Identification: The onchosphere migrating through the liver parenchyma is 5-8.5 mm. long. On entering the peritoneal cavity, the bladderworm lies in a delicate cyst formed from the peritoneum. The vesicle, 5 cm. or more in diameter, contains a watery fluid and the cysticercus with an invaginated scolex.

Distribution and importance: Widely distributed throughout North America; economically important because parts or the whole carcass may be condemned.

Life cycle: The hexacanth embryo hatches in the intestine and migrates to the liver via the portal circulation. It burrows through the liver parenchyma to the surface and enters the peritoneal cavity after about 3-4 weeks. The mature bladder worms may be found anywhere in the peritoneal cavity. The definitive host becomes infected by ingesting the cysticercus.

Transmission: Ingestion of the cysticercus.

Signs and pathogenicity: On reaching the peritoneum the cysticercus is of little pathogenic importance. During the wandering phase of the onchosphere or of the cysticercus through the liver parenchyma, considerable tissue damage, described as hepatitis cysticercosa, may occur. In heavy infections the liver lesions may be extensive, and the hemorrhages may cause death in young animals.

Diagnosis: Usually made at necropsy. Dark red tracks and burrows may be seen on the liver surface, and signs of peritonitis may be present.

Control: Prevention is the easiest means of control. Dogs should be treated regularly, and cysticerci in slaughtered animals should be destroyed. Do not feed sheep offal to dogs unless it is cooked or frozen to kill the cysticerci.

Selected references:

Sweatman, G. K., and P. J. G. Plummer. 1957. The biology and pathology of the tapeworm *Taenia hydatigena* in domestic and wild hosts. *Can. J. Zool.* 35:93-109.

PARASITE: *Davainea proglottina* (minute tapeworm)

Disease: Davaineiasis.

Host: Poultry, pigeons, and other galliform birds.

Habitat: Duodenal loop of small intestine.

Identification: Strobila usually composed of fewer than 9 segments; entire worm is 3-4 mm. long. Rostellum and suckers are armed with several rows of minute hooklets. The spherical egg may be 40 μ in diameter.

Distribution and importance: Widely distributed throughout the U.S.; considered to be highly pathogenic.

Life cycle: Gravid segments are passed in the feces, and eggs hatch after being swallowed by several species of slug. Within the slug, cysticercoids develop in approximately 3 weeks. The prepatent period is about 2 weeks. The eggs containing onchospheres are readily killed by desiccation or freezing.

Transmission: Ingestion of slugs (*Limax*, *Arion*, or *Agriolimax*) containing the cysticercoids.

Signs and pathogenicity: Infected birds show marked emaciation, general debility, and loss of weight. On necropsy the intestinal mucosa appears thickened and may be hemorrhagic because hold-fast organs are heavily armed.

Diagnosis: Demonstration of the cestodes on necropsy by examining mucosal scrapings or by opening the duodenum under water and observing the activity of the papillaelike, minute tapeworms.

Control: Birds free on range are more liable to become infected than those in pens and dry yards. Soil may be treated with metaldehyde to destroy slugs. Pens and range should be well drained. A sandy soil is preferable. Di-n-butyl tin dilaurate is a highly effective treatment agent.

Selected references:

Abdou, A. H. 1956. The use of di-n-butyl tin dilaurate for treatment of chickens experimentally infected with *Davainea proglottina*. *J. Helminthol.* 30:121-28.

Edgar, S. A. 1956. The removal of chicken tapeworms by di-n-butyl tin dilaurate. *Poult. Sci.* 35:64-73.

Levine, P. P. 1938. The effect of infection with *Davainea proglottina* on the weights of growing chickens. *J. Parasitol.* 24:550-51.

PARASITE: *Diphyllobothrium latum* (broad fish tapeworm)

Disease: Diphyllobothriasis.

Host: Man, dog, fox, bear, and other fish-eating mammals.

Habitat: Small intestine.

Identification: One of the longer cestodes; may be 10 meters long and consists of several thousand segments. It is creamy-gray. The scolex is almond-shaped with 2 elongate bothria. The mature segment has a rosette-shaped uterus and a uterine pore. The operculate egg, about $65 \times 40 \mu$, is light brown.

Distribution and importance: Enzootic in the Great Lakes region of North America, found in a small area of Florida and throughout the Arctic. It is historical and aesthetic interest. Of importance in human medicine is its utilization of Vitamin B_{12} at the host's expense and the clinical evidence of pernicious anemia in the human host.

Life cycle: After passing out of the host, the egg develops for several weeks and hatches. A coracidium, an onchosphere (with 6 hooklets) covered with a ciliated embryophore, is then liberated. After ingestion by a suitable crustacean (*Cyclops* or *Diaptomus*), it develops to a procercoid in 2-3 weeks within the body cavity of the crustacean. The infected crustacean is swallowed by the 2nd intermediate host, a fish. The plerocercoid, a solid, larval form, develops in the fish muscle and may be 2 cm. long. The 2nd intermediate host is a pike, trout, salmon, or perch.

Transmission: Ingestion of raw fish containing the plerocercoid.

Signs and pathogenicity: Adult worm is not very pathogenic in the definitive hosts except man. In man the parasite competes with the host for Vitamin B_{12}. Pernicious anemia may result.

Diagnosis: Identification of the operculate egg or gravid segments in the feces of the definitive host.

Control: Prevent ingestion of raw or insufficiently cooked fish. For removal of adults, quinacrine, Yomesan, and arecoline have all proved effective.

Selected references:

Von Bonsdorff, B. 1956. *Diphyllobothrium latum* as a cause of pernicious anemia. *Exp. Parasitol.* 5:207-30.

Weinstein, P. P., and J. G. Appleget. 1952. Some observations on *Diphyllobothrium latum* from Shagwa Lake, Minnesota. *Am. J. Trop. Med. Hyg.* 1:302-06.

PARASITE: *Dipylidium caninum* (double-pored tapeworm)

Disease: Dipylidiasis.
Host: Dog, cat, fox, occasionally child.
Habitat: Small intestine.
Identification: May be 50 cm. long and may be pinkish-red. The rostellum bears 3-4 rows of very small hooks. The mature segment has a genital pore on each lateral margin. The oval gravid segment is elongate and is shaped somewhat like a cucumber seed; it contains egg capsules or packets, each containing as many as 20 eggs.
Distribution and importance: Generally widespread throughout North America.
Life cycle: Involves an intermediate host that may be the dog or cat flea (*Ctenocephalides canis* or *C. felis*) or the louse (*Trichodectes* sp.). Gravid tapeworm segments are passed in the host's feces, and, while warm, the segments move about actively on the stool surface. As the segments dry, they contract and the capsules of eggs are disseminated in the vicinity of the stool. The egg is ingested by the adult louse or the flea larvae. The active onchosphere, 25-30 μ in diameter, develops to the infective cysticercoid stage in the adult arthropod. The definitive host becomes infected by ingesting the infected arthropod. The prepatent period is 2-3 weeks.
Transmission: By ingesting the flea or louse containing an infective cysticercoid.
Signs and pathogenicity: In heavy infections a chronic enteritis may be present. Nervous disturbance and tension are attributed to tapeworm infections and may be associated with such clinical signs as abdominal discomfort, vomiting, convulsions, and severe epileptiform fits. It is thought that tapeworms produce toxic by-products that cause nervous disorders. Gravid segments around the anus may cause anal irritation. This causes "scooting," an attempt to alleviate the anal pruritus.
Diagnosis: Identification of tapeworm segment crawling on the stool or dried on the perianal hairs. Tapeworm eggs or egg packets can be found on fecal examination if segments have been crushed on passage through the anal sphincter or mechanically broken as the feces are stirred or sieved.
Control: Control of fleas and lice. Good sanitation should be maintained in kennels, and insecticides should be used. Many suitable taeniacides are available such as Nemural, Dichlorophen, Scolaban, and Yomesan.

Selected references:

Bradley, R. E. 1971. Tapeworms. In *Current veterinary therapy IV. Small animal practice*, ed. R. W. Kirk, pp. 574-76. Philadelphia: Saunders.
Chen, H. T. 1934. Reactions of *Ctenocephalides felis* to *Dipylidium caninum*. Z. *Parasitenk*. 6:603-37.

PARASITE: *Echinococcus granulosus, E. multilocularis* (hydatid tapeworm)

Disease: Echinococcosis.

Host: *E. granulosus:* dog, jackal, wolf, and other canids. Intermediate hosts are herbivores, and man, pig, and many other mammals. *E. multilocularis:* canids and the domestic cat. Intermediate hosts are microtene rodents such as the vole and lemming; occasionally man is infected.

Habitat: Adults in small intestine. Larval stages are usually in lung and liver; however, any organ may be infected.

Identification: *E. granulosus:* One of the smaller cestodes, 2-5 mm. long. The strobila consists of 3-4 proglottids. The scolex bears 28-46 hooklets arranged in 2 rows. The egg is about 35 by 25 μ. *E. multilocularis:* A small tapeworm, 1.0-3.7 mm. long, of 3-5 segments. The 26-36 hooks are slightly smaller than those of *E. granulosus.*

Distribution and importance: Irregularly enzootic throughout North America. *E. granulosus* is important in areas of intensive sheep production.

Life cycle: The egg is ingested by an intermediate host and hatches in the intestine. The embryo migrates via the bloodstream to various organs, usually liver and lung although almost any organ or tissue may be involved. The intermediate host may be a domestic or wild mammal or, occasionally, man. The embryo develops into a large vesicle, 5-10 cm. in diameter, which is known as an echinococcus or hydatid cyst. A typical cyst has a fairly thick cuticle which is concentrically laminated, and a germinal layer lies on the inside. As it develops, it produces vesicles or brood capsules about 5-6 months after initial infection. Scolices may form from the germinal layer of the brood capsule or from the germinal layer of the mother cyst. Each brood capsule may contain 40 or more scolices. The viability of hydatid cysts in the intermediate hosts is quite variable. In cattle 90% of the cysts may be sterile, in swine about 20%, and in sheep about 8%. The definitive host acquires the infection by ingesting the fertile hydatid cyst in the tissues of the intermediate host. In the dog the prepatent period is 7-9 weeks. In *E. multilocularis* the life cycle, involving a microtene intermediate host, is similar to that of *E. granulosus;* however, the prepatent period is only 4-5 weeks.

Transmission: Ingestion of fertile hydatid cyst in a herbivorous intermediate host.

Signs and pathogenicity: The adult tapeworm in the small intestine of the carnivore seems to be comparatively harmless except if present in large numbers; then an enteritis may develop. Damage caused by the cyst depends on the organ invaded and the size of the cyst. In domestic animals, disease due to hydatids is rare. However, domestic animals are a potential reservoir for infection of carnivores from whom man may become infected.

Diagnosis: Seldom made in the living animal. In man immunodiagnostic tests are widely used. A large cyst fluctuating in size in the liver or lungs may be determined by percussion.

Control: Regular anthelmintic treatment of dogs. All meat or offal fed to dogs and captive carnivores should be inspected and cooked before feeding. Man is usually infected by ingestion of eggs in carnivore feces contaminating hands, leafy vegetables, or fruits. Suitable taeniacides for removal of the adult worms are arecoline hydrobromide, Nemural, Anthelin, Yomesan, and Scolaban.

Selected references:

Araujo, F. P., C. W. Schwabe, J. C. Sawyer, and W. G. Davis. 1975. Hydatid disease transmission in California. A study of the Basque connection. *Am. J. Epidem.* 102:291-302.

Leiby, P. D., and D. C. Kritsky. 1972. *Echinococcus multilocularis:* a possible domestic life cycle in central North America and its public health implications. *J. Parasitol.* 58:1213-15.

Smyth, J. D. 1964. The biology of the hydatid organisms. *Adv. Parasitol.* ed. B. Dawes. 2:169-219.

Sweatman, G. K., and R. J. Williams. 1963. Comparative studies on the biology and morphology of *Echinococcus granulosus* from domestic livestock, moose, and reindeer. *Parasitology* 53:339-90.

PARASITE: *Hymenolepis* spp. (thread tapeworm)

Disease: Hymenolepiasis.

Host: Galliform and anseriform domestic and wild birds, small mammals, and man.

Habitat: Small intestine.

Identification: The genus contains a large number of species that are difficult to identify. The threadlike, fragile strobila is 3-8 cm. long. Generally 3 testes are seen in each mature segment. The egg is large, as large as 80 μ in diameter.

Distribution and importance: Widely distributed throughout North America; not generally considered very important.

Life cycle: A wide variety of intermediate hosts serves the members of the genus. Earwigs, dung beetles, millipedes, fleas, meal moths, grain beetles, and crustaceans may be hosts. The cysticercoid develops in the arthropod intermediate host in 2-3 weeks. The prepatent period is 2-4 weeks.

Transmission: Ingestion of the infective cysticercoid in suitable intermediate host.

Signs and pathogenicity: The sign usually observed in heavily infected birds is growth retardation. Several other signs have inadvertently been attributed to tapeworm infections, often with little supporting evidence.

Diagnosis: The most satisfactory diagnosis is made at necropsy. If the fresh intestine is opened in a small amount of warm water, the worms may be seen actively moving in the water above the mucosal surface. Intestinal scrapings should be examined under the binocular dissecting microscope.

Control: Probably the most important preventive measure in the control of poultry cestodes is proper disposal of droppings. Houses should be cleaned regularly and the manure spread thinly on arable land where sunlight and desiccation will soon destroy the parasitic forms. Numbers of intermediate hosts may be reduced by using insecticides, molluscicides, and other appropriate control measures. The use of medication is somewhat limited for poultry because the cash value of the domestic fowl is usually quite low. Butynorate seems to give the most satisfactory results in the removal of several species of this tapeworm.

Selected references:

Luttermoser, G. W. 1940. The effect on the growth rate of young chickens of infections of the tapeworm, *Hymenolepis carioca. Proc. Helm. Soc. Wash.* 7:74-76.

Mayhew, R. L. 1925. Studies on the avian species of the cestode family Hymenolepididae. *Ill. Biol. Monogr.* 10.

PARASITE: *Moniezia expansa, M. benedeni* (common tapeworm)

Disease: Monieziasis.

Host: *M. expansa:* sheep, goats. *M. benedeni:* ruminants, chiefly cattle.

Habitat: Small intestine.

Identification: *M. expansa:* The creamy-white adult may be 400 cm. long. The suckers are prominent, and segments are broader than long. The interproglottid glands at the posterior border of each segment extend across the width of the segment. The egg is about 60 μ in diameter with a well-developed pyriform apparatus. In *M. benedeni* the interproglottid glands are in a short row close to the center of the posterior border of the segment.

Distribution and importance: Widely distributed; economic importance questionable unless large numbers of tapeworms are present.

Life cycle: The egg is liberated from the expelled gravid tapeworm segment. It is eaten by an oribatid mite that apparently breaks the eggshell and ingests the onchosphere. The young tapeworm grows slowly in the hemocoel of the mite. A cysticercoid containing a scolex is recognizable about 15 weeks after ingestion by the mite. After the infected mite is ingested by the definitive host, the tapeworm matures in about 40 days. The adult lives 2-6 months.

Transmission: By ingestion of infected oribatid mite. In North America numerous species of mites from the following genera serve as suitable intermediate hosts: *Galumna, Oribatula, Peloribates, Protoscheloribates,* and *Scheloribates.*

Signs and pathogenicity: There is considerable disagreement about the pathogenicity of tapeworms in sheep and cattle. Light infections in older animals generally do not cause any trouble. However, massive infections in young lambs cannot be considered harmless. The passage of large masses of gravid segments helps persuade the owner to think seriously about a parasite-control program. Heavy infections in lambs have been reported associated with digestive disturbances, diarrhea, stunted growth, emaciation, wool loss, and anemia.

Diagnosis: Observation of segments in the feces. The segments resemble cooked rice grains. If gravid segments are crushed on passage through the rectum, eggs may be seen on fecal examination.

Control: Avoid permanent pastures. Treat animals and remove them to clean pasture. Copper sulfate, lead arsenate, and dichlorophen are all effective in the removal of this cestode.

Selected references:

Hansen, M. F., A. C. Todd, G. W. Kelley, and M. Cawein. 1950. Effects of a pure infection of the tapeworm *Monieza expansa* in lambs. *Ky. Agr. Expt. Stat. Bul.* 556:3-11.

PARASITE: *Raillietina cesticellus* (broad-headed tapeworm)

Disease: Raillietiniasis.

Host: Domestic fowl.

Habitat: Small intestine, especially duodenum and jejunum.

Identification: The mature worm may be 12 cm. long. The rostellum is armed with 300-500 minute hooks. The egg capsule contains only one egg. The diameter of each egg is 75-85 μ.

Distribution and importance: Generally throughout North America, not recognized as an important pathogen.

Life cycle: The gravid segment passed in the feces is ingested by the intermediate host. Many species of beetles or the house fly may serve. Within the intermediate host, the larval tapeworm becomes infective in 2-4 weeks. The prepatent period is about 3 weeks.

Transmission: Ingestion of the intermediate host containing the cysticercoid.

Signs and pathogenicity: Emaciation and stunted growth have been observed in birds with heavy infections of this cestode. In laying birds, egg production may be decreased or may stop altogether.

Diagnosis: Presence of large numbers of segments or eggs in the feces; demonstration of worms on necropsy.

Control: Control of intermediate hosts with insecticides has been practiced with some success. Removal and disposal of droppings is an important preventive measure. The recommended treatment is di-n-butyl tin dilaurate (Butynorate) or Yomesan in the food.

Selected references:

Edgar, S. A. 1956. The removal of chicken tapeworms by di-n-butyl tin dilaurate. *Poult. Sci.* 35:64-73.

Kerr, K. B. 1952. Butynorate, an effective and safe substance for the removal of *Raillietina cesticellus* from chickens. *Poult. Sci.* 31:328-36.

Reid, W. M., J. E. Ackert, and A. A. Case. 1938. Studies on the life history and biology of the fowl tapeworm, *Raillietina cesticellus. Trans. Amer. Micros. Soc.* 57: 65-76.

PARASITE: *Spirometra mansonoides*

Disease: Spirometriasis.

Host: Cat, occasionally dog.

Habitat: Small intestine.

Identification: Closely resembles species of *Diphyllobothrium*. The egg is more pointed than the *D. latum* egg, and the uterus is a spiral of 2-7 coils rather than a rosette.

Distribution and importance: Reported from scattered areas of the southern U.S., of little economic importance.

Life cycle: First intermediate host is a species of *Cyclops*. The larval stage is referred to as a sparganum or plerocercoid stage and is found in the 2nd intermediate host, a rat, snake, or wild mouse.

Transmission: Ingestion of spargana in tissues of the 2nd intermediate host.

Signs and pathogenicity: The sparganum in man and animals may cause a local indurated area adjacent to the parasite, some urticaria, and occasionally tissue edema. The adult form does not seem to cause any marked lesions.

Diagnosis: Identification of eggs in the feces and of segments passed naturally or as a result of medication.

Control: Prevent ingestion of snakes and small mammals.

Selected references:

Mueller, J. F. 1974. The biology of *Spirometra. J. Parasitol.* 60:3-14.

PARASITE: *Taenia* spp. (armed tapeworms except *T. saginata*)

Disease: Taeniasis.
Host:

Adult	Host	Larval stage	Intermediate host	Habitat
T. saginata	Man	*Cysticercus bovis*	Bovine species	Muscle
T. solium	Man	*Cysticercus cellulosae*	Pig	Muscle
T. hydatigena	Dog	*Cysticercus tenuicollis*	Sheep, cow, pig	Peritoneum
T. krabbei	Dog	*Cysticercus tarandi*	Reindeer	Muscle
T. multiceps	Dog	*Coenurus cerebralis*	Sheep	C.N.S.
T. ovis	Dog	*Cysticercus ovis*	Sheep	Muscle
T. pisiformis	Dog	*Cysticercus pisiformis*	Rabbit	Peritoneum
T. serialis	Dog	*Coenurus serialis*	Rabbit, hare	Connective tissue
T. taeniaformis	Cat	*Cysticercus fasciolaris*	Rat, mouse	Liver

Habitat: Small intestine of definitive host and a variety of organs and tissues in the intermediate host.

Identification: *Taenia* spp. are difficult to differentiate morphologically; specific determination should be left to a specialist. Differential characteristics are the number and size of rostellar hooks and the number of lateral uterine branches in the mature segment. Length may vary from a few inches to several meters. With the exception of *T. saginata*, each species has a rostellum armed with hooks of size and shape characteristic of the species. Each segment has a single set of genitalia; genital pores are single and alternate irregularly. The egg is brown and is about 40 μ in diameter.

Distribution and importance: Widely distributed throughout North America. Adults are important parasites of canids, and larvae are of considerable public health importance and epidemiological significance. As a zoonosis, taeniasis is a veterinary responsibility.

Life cycle: The life cycles of most species are generally similar. Ripe segments are passed in the feces, and the eggs are disseminated on the forage near the fecal mass. The embryophore is ingested, and the onchosphere is liberated in the upper small intestine. By use of its hooklets, it migrates through the mucosa, enters the bloodstream, and is carried to other organs. It develops further when it reaches its preferred tissue. Here it becomes infective 2-3 months after ingestion and remains until consumed by the final host. The prepatent period for most species is 7-8 weeks.

Transmission: The intermediate host is infected by ingesting viable eggs on contaminated forage, food, or utensils. The definitive host acquires the infection by ingesting the larval parasite in muscle or other infected tissues.

Signs and pathogenicity: The adult tapeworms are not usually spectacular pathogens unless large numbers cause intestinal obstruction. The importance of these species lies in the epidemiology of the larval forms. Onchospheres and developing cysticerci may cause severe damage when migrating through the liver tissue. Such a condition is sometimes termed hepatitis cysticercosa.

Diagnosis: Presence of tapeworm segments in the feces or, if segments have been broken on passage through the rectum or by mechanical rupture, eggs may be demonstrated on fecal examination.

Control: Regular treatment of dogs for tapeworms and destruction of cysticerci recovered from slaughtered intermediate hosts. If offal is fed to dogs, cysticerci should be killed by freezing or cooking. Taeniacides such as nemural, dichlorophen, bunamidine, and niclosamide are effective. To prevent human infections of *Taenia*, dressed meat should be inspected and adequately cooked before consumption.

Selected references:

Pawlowski, Z., and M. G. Schultz. 1972. *Taeniasis and cysticercosis (T. saginata)*. *Adv. Parasitol.* ed. B. Dawes. 10:269-343.

PARASITE: *Thysanosoma actinoides* (fringed tapeworm)

Disease: Thysanosomiasis.

Host: Sheep, goats, deer, and other wild ruminants.

Habitat: Small intestine and the biliary system, frequently congregated at the opening of the common bile duct into the duodenum and in the distal end of the common duct.

Identification: To 30 cm. long; segments are short and fringed posteriorly. A double set of genital organs is found in each segment. Several paruterine organs are formed in each segment in which multiple onchospheres develop. Eggs do not have a pyriform apparatus.

Distribution and importance: Limited largely to the western states of the U.S.; causes appreciable economic loss resulting from condemnation of livers. Otherwise losses are slight.

Life cycle: Complete life history still unknown. Developmental stages including the cysticercoid have been recovered from several species of psocids (barklice), but attempts to infect sheep by feeding cysticercoids from psocids have not been successful.

Transmission: Incompletely known, probably by infected psocid mites.

Signs and pathogenicity: No definite clinical signs have been attributed to this parasite. Some inflammation of the biliary epithelium has been observed. Enlargement of the bile duct with marked fibrosis and hyperplasia of the wall may be seen. The tapeworm does not appear to have any negative effect on growth rate of lambs.

Diagnosis: Demonstration of segments on fecal pellets is the most valuable diagnostic tool.

Control: Acquisition of fringed tapeworm on open range seems to be a seasonal phenomenon, occurring in late summer and early winter. Lambs should be moved from range to irrigated pastures or feedlots before the tapeworm transmission begins. Anthelmintics of choice are bithionol, Yomesan, and cambendazole.

Selected references:

Allen, R. W. 1973. The biology of *Thysanosoma actinoides*, a parasite of domestic and wild animals. *N. M. State University, Agr. Expt. Station Bul.* 604.

Allen, R. W., F. D. Enzie, and K. S. Samson. 1962. Effects of bithionol and other compounds on the fringed tapeworm, *Thysanosoma actinoides* in sheep. *Am. J. Vet. Res.* 23:236-40.

C. Trematodes

Disease: Alariasis.

Host: Dog. Various carnivores serve as hosts for other species.

Habitat: Small intestine, often in duodenum.

Identification: To 6 mm. long and about 2 mm. wide. At each side of the anterior end is a small earlike structure that is helpful in identification. The golden-brown egg is large, to 134 μ long and about 70 μ wide, and contains circular granular structures. The cercaria has a bifurcate tail.

Distribution and importance: Essentially nonpathogenic as far as is known. However, the eggs are frequently seen on flotation fecal examination and may cause the veterinarian some concern.

Life cycle: The egg hatches in about 2 weeks, and the miracidium penetrates a freshwater snail of the genus *Helisoma*. The cercaria is shed by the snail and then penetrates a 2nd intermediate host such as a tadpole or frog. This larval stage is called a mesocercaria, similar to the metacercaria in other flukes. The final host may become infected by ingesting the amphibian containing the mesocercaria. The larval fluke migrates through the abdominal and thoracic cavities to the lung, trachea, and pharynx and finally reaches the small intestine. Apparently the 2nd intermediate host may be ingested by another animal such as a mouse, rat, snake, or bird. These serve as paratenic hosts and are a source of infective flukes if eaten by the definitive host.

Transmission: Ingestion of the infected intermediate host or one of the many paratenic hosts.

Signs and pathogenicity: Members of this genus are not considered pathogenic, though a catarrhal duodenitis has been attributed to heavy infections. A fatal human infection with mesocercariae of *A. americana* has been reported.

Diagnosis: Identification of large, golden-brown, operculate eggs.

Control: Treatment or other types of control are seldom attempted. Yomesan or bithionol might be tried if treatment is indicated.

Selected references:

Freeman, R. S., P. F. Stuart, J. B. Cullen, A. C. Ritchie, A. Mildon, B. J. Fernandes, and R. Bonin. 1976. Fatal human infection with mesocercariae of the trematode *Alaria americana. Am. J. Trop. Med. Hyg.* 25:803-07.

Hayden, D. W. 1969. Alariasis in a dog. *J. Am. Vet. Med. Assoc.* 155:889-91.

Pearson, J. C. 1956. Studies on the life cycle and morphology of the larval stages of *Alaria arisaemoides* Augustine and Uribe, 1927, and *Alaria canis* LaRue and Fallis, 1936. *Can. J. Zool.* 34:295-387.

PARASITE: *Collyriclum faba* (skin fluke)

Disease: Collyriclumiasis.

Host: Chicken, turkey, and wild birds.

Habitat: Encysted in the skin, frequently in the region of the cloaca and vent.

Identification: Parasites frequently found in pairs within a subcutaneous cyst. The fluke is plump and spiny, to 8 mm. long and 5 mm. wide. The oral sucker is terminal, and there is no acetabulum. The egg is about 20 x 10 μ. The cyst containing the fluke is usually 4-6 mm. in diameter.

Distribution and importance: In the U.S., reported only from Minnesota. The cysts greatly depreciate infected birds and probably are sufficient cause for carcass condemnation. However, the restricted distribution of this parasite renders it of limited economic importance.

Life cycle: Life history of the fluke is unknown. It is reasonable to assume that the 1st intermediate host is a snail and the 2nd intermediate host is probably an arthropod. Metacercarial forms resembling the adult have been found in dragonfly nymphs, and infection seems to be most common in birds having access to marshy places.

Transmission: Unknown.

Signs and pathogenicity: Skin surface in region of cloaca and vent may be badly soiled by a black fluid discharged through the cyst pore.

Diagnosis: Demonstration of flukes or fluke eggs from subcutaneous cysts.

Control: Keep birds away from swampy, wet areas.

Selected references:

Riley, W. A. 1931. *Collyriclum faba* as a parasite of poultry. *Poult. Sci.* 10:204-07.

Riley, W. A., and H. C. H. Kernkamp. 1924. Flukes of the genus *Collyriclum* as parasites of turkeys and chickens. *J. Amer. Vet. Med. Assoc.* 64:591-99.

PARASITE: *Dicrocoelium dendriticum* (lancet fluke)

Disease: Dicrocoeliasis.

Host: Cattle, sheep, goats, and many other mammals such as rabbits, deer, and occasionally man.

Habitat: Bile ducts, gall bladder.

Identification: Small, transparent, lanceolate fluke to 10 mm. long and 2.5 mm. wide. The cuticle is smooth. The brown, operculate egg is about 40 x 25 μ. The prepatent period is 11-12 weeks.

Distribution and importance: New York and Pennsylvania, as yet not of major importance in the U.S.

Life cycle: The miracidium hatches after the egg is swallowed by the molluscan intermediate host *Cionella lubrica*. The sporocyst develops and produces cercariae in about 3 months. The snail produces slime balls, each containing many cercariae. On being expelled from the snail, the slime ball adheres to vegetation and is ingested by an ant of the genus *Formica*. The metacercaria develops in the abdominal cavity of the ant, and the definitive host becomes infected by swallowing infected ants. The metacercaria penetrates the intestinal wall of the definitive host and reaches the bile ducts by way of the portal circulation or by entering the intestinal opening of the common bile duct.

Transmission: Ingestion of infected ants.

Signs and pathogenicity: Not usually marked except in very severe infections in which extensive hepatic cirrhosis and distention of the bile ducts occur. Bile duct eipthelium and fibroblasts may proliferate. The liver may appear lumpy and scarred owing to the greatly distended bile ducts. Anemia, edema, emaciation, and loss of condition may be seen.

Diagnosis: Identification of the egg containing a miracidium on fecal examination or of the adult on necropsy.

Control: Chemical or biological control is difficult. Eggs of the fluke may withstand freezing and remain viable in the soil over long periods. Land snails are less vulnerable to molluscicides than are water snails, and in the U.S. such animals as the woodchuck may serve as reservoir hosts for the flukes. Treatment with Hetolin gives good results. Thiabendazole at high dosage levels has been found effective.

Selected references:

Krull, W. H., and C. R. Mapes. 1953. Studies on the biology of *Dicrocoelium dendriticum* including its relation to the intermediate host, *Cionella lubrica*. IX. Notes on the cyst, metacercariae and infection in the ant *Formica fusca*. *Cornell Vet.* 43:389-410.

Sinclair, K. B. 1967. Pathogenesis of *Fasciola* and other liver flukes. *Helminthol. Abstr.* 36:115-34.

PARASITE: *Echinostoma revolutum*

Disease: Echinostomiasis.

Host: Chicken, duck, turkey, many other wild birds, and some mammals.

Habitat: Intestine, ceca, cloaca.

Identification: Flukes have a kidney-shaped collar (adoral disc) armed with 1 or 2 rows of spines. Body is elongate, to 22 mm. long. The egg is about 110 by 65 μ.

Distribution and importance: Widely distributed throughout North America but does not appear to be an important pathogen.

Life cycle: Many species of freshwater snails can serve as the 1st intermediate host. The cercaria usually encysts in a 2nd intermediate host that is a snail or a tadpole. The final host becomes infected by ingesting the infected snail or tadpole. The prepatent period is about 12 days.

Transmission: Ingestion of an infected 2nd intermediate host.

Signs and pathogenicity: In light infections these flukes cause little injury. If large numbers are present, it is claimed they may cause severe enteritis, hemorrhagic diarrhea, and progressive emaciation.

Diagnosis: Identification of eggs in the feces or adult worms in the intestine on necropsy examination.

Control: Avoid wet marsh areas. Snail control should be considered.

Selected references:

Kitchell, R. L., J. S. Cass, and J. H. Sautter. 1947. An infestation in domestic turkeys with intestinal flukes. *J. Amer. Vet. Med. Assoc.* 111:379-81.

PARASITE: *Faciola hepatica* (common liver fluke)

Disease: Fascioliasis.

Host: Sheep, goat, cattle, and occasionally horse and swine.

Habitat: Bile ducts, gall bladder. Occasionally it is found in the lungs and elsewhere in aberrant hosts.

Identification: May be 30 mm. or longer. The greyish-brown adult is leaf-shaped, broader anteriorly than posteriorly. The anterior end bears a cone-shaped projection and a pair of "broad shoulders." The cuticle is armed with spines. The intestinal ceca are branched as are the testes and the ovary. Vitelline follicles fill the lateral fields of the worm, and the uterus extends through the midportion to the common genital pore just anterior to the acetabulum. The egg is about 140 x 75 μ and has an operculum not always easily seen.

Distribution and importance: Widely reported throughout North America; economic importance is associated primarily with condemnation of cattle livers containing flukes.

Life cycle: The egg passes down the bile duct to the intestine and out with the droppings. Development and hatching depend on temperature. If there is sufficient moisture, eggs will hatch in 2-3 weeks at usual summer temperatures (25°C.). The miracidium is ciliated, has a pair of eye spots, and develops further only after finding an appropriate lymnaeid snail. Intermediate hosts may be *Lymnaea truncatula, L. bulimoides techella, L. palustris,* and *L. stagnalis.* Within the snail the miracidium sheds its cilia and becomes a sporocyst, about 1 mm. long. The sporocyst reproduces asexually producing several redia which ultimately produce cercariae. Depending on temperature and rate of development, the cercaria is shed by the snail 5-7 weeks after initial penetration of the miracidium. The cercaria swims to a firm surface, usually plant material such as a blade of grass or a piece of leaf. It encysts and is then known as a metacercaria, infective to the mammalian host. The metacercaria may be 2 mm. in diameter.

After ingestion by a mammal, excystation occurs in the duodenum and the immature fluke finds its way to the body cavity. The fluke usually has penetrated the liver capsule and is found migrating through the liver parenchyma 4-6 days after infection. Some flukes are thought to reach the liver by way of the bloodstream.

Transmission: By ingestion of metacercariae.

Signs and pathogenicity: Dependent on number of metacercariae ingested. A traumatic hepatitis may develop owing to the migration of large numbers of immature flukes. Severe destruction of liver parenchyma with marked hemorrhage may occur. The animal may die several days after the appearance of the initial signs of anorexia and immobility. The acute form of the disease, less common than the chronic form, may be complicated by the condition known as "black disease" caused by *Clostridium novyi.* In the chronic form of the disease rather vague signs such as general debility, emaciation, depression, and lack of vigor with anemia, pale mucosae, and submaxillary edema are characteristic.

Diagnosis: Demonstration of eggs in the feces or recovery of flukes at necropsy.

Control: Consists of attacking the flukes in the liver and eliminating the snail intermediate host. Many new fasciolicides are available, though an old standby for treating sheep is carbon tetrachloride. Hexachloroethane is used to treat sheep and cattle. Infection may be prevented by avoiding wet pastures and not using hay from infected pastures. Pastures may be drained, and a molluscicide, 1:500,000 copper sulfate, may be applied to wet areas. Copper sulfate dust may be broadcast over snail habitats at the rate of 10-30 lb. per acre depending on the type of water surface to be treated. Copper pentachlorophenate is another apparently effective molluscicide. For the alleviation of black disease, a vaccine against *C. novyi* is available.

Selected references:

Armour, J. 1975. The epidemiology and control of bovine fascioliasis. *Vet. Rec.* 96: 198-201.
Ollerenshaw, C. B. 1959. The ecology of the liver fluke. *Vet. Rec.* 71:957-65.
Sinclair, K. B. 1967. Pathogenesis of *Fasciola* and other liver flukes. *Helminthol. Abstr.* 36:115-34.
Taylor, E. L. 1964. Fascioliasis and the liver fluke. *F.A.O. Agr. Studies No. 4.*
Turner, A. W. 1930. Black disease (Infectious necrotic hepatitis) of sheep in Australia. *C.S.I.R.O. (Australia) Bull. 46.*

PARASITE: *Fascioloides magna* (large American fluke)

Disease: Fascioloidiasis.

Host: Deer, cattle, sheep, and pig.

Habitat: Liver parenchyma and occasionally other organs such as the lung.

Identification: A large, fleshy, oval fluke to 7-5 cm. long and 3 cm. wide. Unlike *F. hepatica* there is no anterior cone, and there are no shoulders. The egg is similar to that of *F. hepatica*; it is operculate and may be 170 μ long and 100 μ wide.

Distribution and importance: Indigenous to North America especially in the Great Lakes region, the Gulf region, the Rocky Mountain states and parts of Canada. It is of considerable importance where sheep and deer use common pastures.

Life cycle: Similar to that of *Fasciola hepatica*. The egg hatches after about 4 weeks. The cercaria develops for 7-8 weeks in a snail intermediate host such as *Stagnicola palustris*, *S. caperata*, *Fossaria parva*, *F. modicella*, and *Lymnaea bulimoides techella*. After the cercaria is liberated, it becomes a metacercaria encysted on vegetation.

Transmission: Ingestion of metacercariae with food and water.

Signs and pathogenicity: Pathogenicity varies with the host. In the Cervidae the host develops a fibrous cyst with thin walls. Both afferent and efferent bile ducts are patent in these hosts, thus the egg of *F. magna* is passed to the outside with the feces. In the Bovidae a closed cyst is produced with a thick fibrous wall which occludes both afferent and efferent bile ducts. The egg is usually not liberated from these hosts. Larger bovine species are unsuitable hosts for this parasite and play no major role in the dissemination of the fluke. The sheep is also an unsuitable host; its reaction to the presence of the fluke is not remarkable. The fluke migrates through the liver parenchyma without encountering host resistance, and a series of necrotic, hemorrhagic tracts is produced. The fluke may reach maturity in the sheep, but usually the host succumbs because the uncontrolled migration of a few parasites results in extensive tissue destruction. The black streaking and pigmentation of tissues accompanying *F. magna* infections is due to regurgitation by the fluke of ingested cellular debris and iron porphyrin. The pigmentation may be seen throughout the liver parenchyma, hepatic and mesenteric lymph nodes, and occasionally throughout the omentum. It would seem reasonable that the tissue destruction by *F. magna* during its hepatic migration in cattle and sheep would provide a suitable situation for the development of *Clostridium novyi* and the occurrence of black disease.

Diagnosis: *F. magna* eggs from infected deer may be demonstrated on fecal examination. In cattle and sheep, diagnosis is made at necropsy by finding flukes or the characteristic black pigmentation throughout the liver parenchyma, hepatic nodes, and other tissues.

Control: Prevention of infection may be attempted by using management programs to reduce snail populations by drainage, fencing, and other procedures. Copper sulfate may be applied to wet areas at the rate of 28 lb. per acre. To aid distribution, the chemical is usually mixed with 4 parts of sand. Prevention might be achieved by excluding deer from cattle and sheep pastures, but this is not easily accomplished. Treatment for mature flukes presents a problem because a fibrous connective tissue cyst surrounds the fluke. It appears that rafoxinide may prove of value as a therapeutic agent.

Selected references:

Foreyt, W. J., and A. C. Todd. 1976. Development of the large American liver fluke, *Fascioloides magna*, in white-tailed deer, cattle and sheep. *J. Parasitol.* 62:26-32.

Griffiths, H. J. 1962. Fascioloidiasis of cattle, sheep and deer in northern Minnesota. *J. Am. Vet. Med. Assoc.* 140:342-47.

Swales, W. E. 1935. The life cycle of *Fascioloides magna* (Bassi, 1875), the large liver fluke of ruminants in Canada. *Can. J. Res.* 12:177-215.

PARASITE: *Heterobilharzia americana* (blood fluke)

Disease: Heterobilharziasis, canine schistosomiasis, water dermatitis.

Host: A wide range of hosts including the dog, nutria, and raccoon.

Habitat: Mesenteric veins of small and large intestines and probably the portal veins.

Identification: The adult fluke is small; the slender female may be as long as 9 mm. The thin-shelled egg, about 80 x 50 μ, has no spine and contains a miracidium. The male worm is about 6.5 mm. long; the postacetabular region is folded in to form the gynaecophoric canal.

Distribution and importance: Limited distribution and economic importance. It is enzootic in the coastal swamplands of Louisiana and the mud flats of the Mississippi delta.

Life cycle: Eggs hatch immediately after deposition if they contact water. The miracidium enters an intermediate host, *Lymnaea cubensis* or *Pseudosuccinea columnella*. The mature cercaria is produced in about 25 days. It penetrates the skin of the mammalian host, finds its way to the lung, thence to the liver and the mesenteric veins. The prepatent period appears to be about 84 days.

Transmission: Contact with water contaminated with cercariae.

Signs and pathogenicity: Infected animals show a marked urticaria with pustular-maculopapular eruptions. An intermittent diarrhea and mucus in the feces seem related to the number of eggs discharged. Infected dogs have been reported to show emaciation, anorexia, and diarrhea and to develop a terminal coma accompanied by bloody diarrhea.

Diagnosis: Identification of eggs in feces.

Control: Restrict access to marsh lands and swampy areas. Treatment is not usually attempted; calamine or a similar medication may alleviate the pruritus.

Selected references:

Malek, E. A., L. R. Ash, H. F. Lee, and M. D. Little. 1961. *Heterobilharzia* infection in the dog and other mammals in Louisiana. *J. Parasitol.* 47:619-23.

Pierce, K. R. 1963. *Heterobilharzia americana* infection in a dog. *J. Am. Vet. Med. Assoc.* 143:496-99.

Thrasher, K. R. 1964. Canine schistosomiasis. *J. Am. Vet. Med. Assoc.* 144:1119-26.

PARASITE: *Metorchis conjunctus*

Disease: Metorchiasis.

Host: Dog, cat, fox, raccoon, and mink.

Habitat: Bile ducts.

Identification: May be 6.6 mm. long and 2.6 mm. wide. The cuticle is usually spiny. The yellow-brown egg may be 32 μ long and 18 μ wide and has a distinct operculum.

Distribution and importance: Of importance in working sled dogs in the northern part of the continent; widely distributed throughout North America.

Life cycle: The egg is ingested by the freshwater snail *Amnicola limnosa porata*. The cercaria from the snail enters the lateral musculature of the common sucker, *Catostomus commersonii*, and the carnivorous host becomes infected by ingesting infected fish muscle. The metacercaria in the fish will survive freezing.

Transmission: Ingestion of infected muscle of the sucker.

Signs and pathogenicity: The trematode may cause a catarrhal cholecystitis, proliferation of the biliary epithelium, and some cirrhosis of liver tissue.

Diagnosis: Confirmed by identifying eggs from the feces.

Control: Raw sucker should not be fed to dogs.

Selected references:

Cameron, T. W. M. C. 1944. The morphology, taxonomy and life history of *Metorchis conjunctus* (Cobbold, 1860). *Can. J. Res.* 22:6-16.

Jordan, H. E., and W. T. Ashby. 1957. Liver fluke (*Metorchis conjunctus*) in a dog from South Carolina. *J. Am. Vet. Med. Assoc.* 131:239-40.

Mills, J. H. L., and R. S. Hirth. 1968. Lesions caused by the hepatic trematode, *Metorchis conjunctus*, Cobbold, 1860: A comparative study in carnivora. *J. Sm. An. Pract.* 9:1-6.

PARASITE: *Nanophyetus salmincola* (Syn: *Troglotrema salmincola*) (salmon-poisoning fluke)

Disease: Nanophyetiasis.

Host: Dog, mink, and other fish-eating mammals. The 1st intermediate host is a snail; the 2nd is a fish of the family Salmonidae.

Habitat: Small intestine, especially duodenum.

Identification: A minute, creamy-white trematode, 0.5-1.1 mm. long. The yellow-brown egg is about 70 x 40 μ and has an indistinct operculum.

Distribution and importance: Enzootic to the Pacific Northwest of North America. This trematode serves as a vector for *Neorickettsia helminthoeca* which is responsible for a severe and often fatal enteritis, so-called salmon poisoning, in dogs. The flukes also transmit the rickettsia associated with Elokomin fluke fever.

Life cycle: The egg is passed in the feces of the carnivorous host and hatches in about 3 months depending on temperature. The miracidium penetrates the snail intermediate host *Oxytrema plicifera*. The cercaria develops, is liberated, and penetrates the 2nd intermediate host, a fish of the family Salmonidae. The metacercaria is found in the muscle, kidney, eye, and other organs and tissues of the fish. The metacercaria is 175-225 μ in diameter and is readily killed by freezing.

Transmission: Ingestion of infected tissues of members of the Salmonidae.

Signs and pathogenicity: Salmon poisoning of carnivores is commonly fatal. Six to ten days after ingestion of infected fish, victims show pronounced fever and complete loss of appetite. This is followed by a purulent eye discharge, vomiting, and profuse diarrhea. Mortality is 50-90%; recovered animals are immune.

Diagnosis: A history of eating appropriate fish followed by the pathognomonic signs of the disease in an animal from the Pacific Northwest provides the basis of diagnosis.

Control: Do not permit access to salmon in enzootic areas. The infection may be successfully treated with tetracycline and serum therapy.

Selected references:

Cordy, R. D., and J. R. Gorham. 1950. The pathology and etiology of salmon disease in the dog and fox. *Am. J. Pathol.* 26:617-37.

Farrell, R. K., R. W. Leader, and S. D. Johnston. 1973. Differentiation of salmon poisoning disease and Elokomin fluke fever; studies with the black bear (*Ursus americanus*). *Am. J. Vet. Res.* 34:919-22.

Hadlow, W. J. 1957. Neuropathology of experimental poisoning of dogs. *Am. J. Vet. Res.* 18:898-908.

Philip, C. B., W. J. Hadlow, and L. E. Hughes. 1954. Studies on salmon poisoning disease of canines. 1. The rickettsial relationship and pathogenicity of *Neorickettsia helminthoeca*. *Expt. Parasitol.* 3:336-50.

PARASITE: *Paragonimus kellicotti* (lung fluke)

Disease: Paragonimiasis.

Host: Cat, dog, mink, and other carnivores. Intermediate hosts are snails and crayfish.

Habitat: Cysts in lung parenchyma, usually 2 or 3 flukes per cyst. Occasionally it may be found in brain and other organs.

Identification: The brownish-red adult may be 16 x 8 mm. long; the cuticle is covered with spines. The yellow-brown egg, about 90 x 50 μ, has an operculum, and the shell at the opposite pole is somewhat thickened.

Distribution and importance: Widely distributed throughout North America; not usually very important in lung tissue.

Life cycle: The egg is laid in the cyst in which the worm lives. The egg is carried to the .bronchus, coughed up in a rusty colored sputum, and passed out in the feces. The miracidium develops in 2-7 weeks and penetrates a snail (*Pomatiopsis lapidaria*). The cercaria develops, is released, and penetrates a crayfish in which it encysts. The definitive host is infected by eating an infected crayfish or drinking water containing a metacercaria that has escaped from the intermediate host. The metacercaria remains viable in water for 3 weeks. After liberation in the intestine of the definitive host, the young fluke penetrates the intestinal wall, wanders through the peritoneal cavity and diaphragm, and enters the lung from the pleural cavity.

Transmission: Ingestion of an infected intermediate host or metacercaria that has been released from the crayfish.

Signs and pathogenicity: A small number of parasites in the lung causes little damage. If the flukes wander to the brain or other vital tissues, they may cause a significant problem. The parasitic cyst is surrounded by connective tissue and is infiltrated with leucocytes and giant cells. The egg provokes a mild reaction, the formation of small pseudotubercles.

Diagnosis: Identification of eggs from sputum or feces.

Control: Do not feed raw crustaceans to dogs or cats. Snail control may be considered. Bithionol acetate has been shown to be effective in the treatment of both man and the dog.

Selected references:

Greve, J. H. 1969. Bithionol treatment of canine paragonimiasis. *J. Am. An. Hosp. Assoc.* 5:118-23.

Greve, J. H., E. D. Roberts, and M. W. Sloss. 1963-64. *Paragonimus* in Iowa. *I. S. U. Vet.* 26:21-28.

Macy, D. W., and K. S. Todd. 1975. Treatment of canine paragonimiasis with bithionol acetate. *Vet. Med. Sm. An. Clin.* 70:57-58.

Majure, T. V., and W. J. Moore. 1975. Clinical observations on lung flukes in the cat. *Vet. Med. Sm. An. Clin.* 70:852-53.

PARASITE: *Paramphistomum* spp. (rumen fluke), *Cotylophoron* sp.

Disease: Paramphistomiasis.

Host: *Paramphistomum* spp.: cattle. *Cotylophoron* sp.: sheep, goat.

Habitat: Rumen, reticulum.

Identification: The adult *Cotylophoron* is morphologically very similar to *Paramphistomum*. Living flukes are cone-shaped or pear-shaped and frequently are light red. They may be 5-13 mm. long and 2-5 mm. wide. These flukes characteristically have a large posterior, subterminal sucker in addition to the oral sucker. The taxonomy of the group is complex and controversial. The egg is about 120-170 x 75-80 μ.

Distribution and importance: Widespread. Immature forms are of major importance; adult flukes seem to be of little significance.

Life cycle: These species have similar life cycles and involve a wide variety of snail intermediate hosts. Some of the common species of aquatic snails are

Lymnaea bulimoides techella, Planorbis sp., *Pseudosuccinea columella, Fossaria modicella,* and *F. parva.* Metacercariae are ingested with food and water, and after 6-8 weeks migration adult flukes may be found in the rumen. The prepatent period is 3-4 months.

Transmission: Ingestion of viable metacercariae with food or water.

Signs and pathogenicity: Infected animals lose appetite and condition. They appear dull and show considerable weakness and signs of anemia. Adult flukes do not seem to be pathogenic. The immature forms are a significant irritant to the intestinal mucosa especially of the duodenum. A catarrhal or hemorrhagic enteritis may occur throughout the upper small intestine.

Diagnosis: Necropsy and demonstration of the adult or immature stages in the digestive tract.

Control: Fence off or drain wet, potentially contaminated areas. Many therapeutic agents have yielded variable results, usually limited effectiveness. Hexachloroethane bentonite seems most promising, though tetrachlorethylene, hexachlorophene, and bithionol have all been recommended.

Selected references:

Boray, J. C. 1959. Studies on intestinal amphistomiasis in cattle. *Aust. Vet. J.* 35: 282-87.

Horak, I. G. 1971. Paramphistomiasis of domestic ruminants. *Adv. Parasitol.* ed. B. Dawes. 9:33-72.

Olsen, O. W. 1949. Action of hexachloroethane bentonite suspension on the rumen fluke, *Paramphistomum. Vet. Med.* 44:108-09.

PARASITE: *Platynosomum concinnum* (Syn.: *P. fastosum*) (cat liver fluke)

Disease: Platynosomiasis.

Host: Cat.

Habitat: Gall bladder, bile ducts.

Identification: Mature fluke is ovoid to lanceolate, to 8.0 mm. long and 2.5 mm. wide. The brownish egg, about 30 x 25 μ, has a thick shell.

Distribution and importance: Most commonly seen in the southern U.S. In enzootic areas it is considered important.

Life cycle: The snail intermediate host *Subulina octona* becomes infected by ingesting the fluke egg. The miracidium emerges in the digestive tract, enters the snail's tissues, and becomes a mother sporocyst. On maturing, daughter sporocysts leave the snail, and a lizard, *Anolis cristatellus,* serves as the 2nd intermediate host. The cat becomes infected by eating the lizard.

Transmission: Ingestion of the infected 2nd intermediate host, the lizard.

Signs and pathogenicity: Vomition, diarrhea, and general emaciation have been attributed to heavy infections of this fluke. On necropsy the liver may be enlarged, and the parasitized bile ducts may show some fibrosis. Hyperplasia of the biliary epithelium has also been observed. Fatal infections have been reported.

Diagnosis: The operculate egg may be demonstrated by use of an egg-flotation procedure or by an ether-sedimentation technique.

Control: No satisfactory treatment is known. Avoid ingesting lizards.

Selected references:

Greve, J. H., and P. O. Leonard. 1966. Hepatic flukes (*Platynosomum concinnum*) in a cat from Illinois. *J. Am. Vet. Med. Assoc.* 149:418-20.

Palumbo, N. E., S. F. Perri, B. Loo, D. Taylor, and V. Reece. 1974. Cat liver fluke, *Platynosomum concinnum*, in Hawaii. *Am. J. Vet. Res.* 35:1455.

PARASITE: *Prosthogonimus macrorchis* (oviduct fluke)

Disease: Prosthogonimiasis.

Host: Domestic fowl and wild birds.

Habitat: Oviduct, bursa of Fabricus.

Identification: Pyriform body, to 7 mm. long, is covered with spines. Numerous eggs are produced. Each thin-shelled egg is about 28 x 16 μ and contains an embryo when laid.

Distribution and importance: Mostly found in the lake regions of Minnesota and Michigan. It is not of major economic significance and probably is important only to the individual who encounters a fluke in an egg.

Life cycle: Two intermediate hosts are necessary, an aquatic snail (*Amnicola* sp.) and a dragonfly. The snail ingests the fluke egg containing a miracidium. Sporocysts develop, but there is no redia stage. The cercariae are liberated from the snail, swim around, and are drawn into the anal opening of a dragonfly naiad as the insect breathes. Within the naiad they become metacercariae.

Transmission: By ingestion of an infected naiad or adult dragonfly.

Signs and pathogenicity: In the young bird, the immature fluke is liberated from the encysted metacercaria and passes to the bursa of Fabricius where it matures. In the older bird, the young fluke enters the oviduct and is markedly pathogenic. An infected bird becomes inactive and loses its appetite. Egg production drops, and those eggs produced have thin shells or no shells at all. On necropsy emaciation, anemia, and a pronounced hyperemia of the intestine may be observed. Rupture of the oviduct may occur with resultant peritonitis.

Diagnosis: Identification of adult flukes on necropsy or of large numbers of fluke eggs in the cloacal discharge.

Control: Limit access of birds to wet, marshy land where dragonflies are commonly found. Snail control may also be practiced. No satisfactory treatment is known.

Selected references:

Kotlan, A., and W. L. Chandler. 1925. A newly recognized fluke disease (prosthogonimiasis) of fowls in the United States. *J. Amer. Vet. Med. Assoc.* 67:756-63.

Macy, R. W. 1934. Studies on the taxonomy, morphology and biology of *Prosthogonimus macrorchis* Macy, a common oviduct fluke of domestic fowl in North America. *Univ. Minn. Agr. Exper. Sta. Bul.* 98:1-71.

D. Acanthocephalans

PARASITE: *Macracanthorhynchus hirudinaceus* (thorny-headed worm, acanthocephalid)

Disease: Porcine acanthocephaliasis.

Host: Pig.

Habitat: Small intestine.

Identification: Pseudosegmented appearance and often pale reddish. The adult may be 35 mm. long or more and 4-10 mm. wide; the cuticle is transversely wrinkled. A small proboscis extends from the anterior end and bears about 6 rows of transverse hooks. The egg is 100 x 65 μ and has 4 shells; the 2nd is brown and pitted.

Distribution and importance: Generally found throughout the central and southern U.S. Its major significance is the damage to intestine that otherwise would be used for casings.

Life cycle: The adult attaches to the intestinal mucosa by a thorny proboscis. The egg passes in the droppings and hatches after ingestion by the intermediate host, a scarabeid dung beetle or a June beetle. The young worm becomes encysted in the body cavity of the beetle after 2 or 3 months. The hog becomes infected by ingesting the infected larval or adult beetle. The prepatent period is 2-3 months.

Transmission: Ingestion of infected June or dung beetles.

Signs and pathogenicity: Using the proboscis, the thorny-heads penetrate deeply into the intestinal mucosa. Perforation may occur with resultant peritonitis. A zone of inflammation may be seen at the point of attachment, which eventually becomes a healed scar. The serosal surface of the small intestine may have greenish-yellow to dark brown nodules the size of a pea at the point of attachment of the worm. Clinical signs are only seen in severe infections and may include digestive disorders, emaciation, and diarrhea.

Diagnosis: Identification of eggs on fecal examination.

Control: Reduce ingestion of infective intermediate hosts by using bare lots or slat or concrete flooring. Heavily contaminated pastures and dirt pens should be abandoned for at least 3 years. Plowing and allowing pasture to lie fallow in summer will help clear the land of contamination. No satisfactory treatment is available.

PARASITE: *Oncicola canis* (thorny-headed worm)

Disease: Oncicoliasis.

Host: Dog.

Habitat: Small intestine.

Identification: A small worm, to 14 mm. long. The body tapers posteriorly, is dark gray, and ends anteriorly in a characteristic proboscis armed with hooks. The brown egg is oval, about 65 x 45 μ.

Distribution and importance: Southern U.S., seldom of clinical importance.

Life cycle: Not fully known, probably an arthropod is involved. Immature forms, about 4 mm. long, have been found encysted in the connective tissue and muscles of the armadillo, which may serve as a 2nd intermediate host or as a paratenic host.

Transmission: Possibly acquired through ingestion of infective tissues of the armadillo. It is more likely that an arthropod intermediate host is involved.

Signs and pathogenicity: The proboscis of the worm is deeply embedded in the intestinal wall. If it penetrates the wall, a peritonitis may occur. Heavy infections have been associated with rabiform signs in the dog.

Diagnosis: Finding the acanthocephalan eggs in the feces.

Control: No known treatment or means of control.

PART III
ARTHROPODS

Arthropods

A. Arachnids

PARASITE: *Argas persicus* (Fowl tick, blue bug)

Disease/Infestation: Argasid acariasis.

Host: Chicken, turkey, and wild birds.

Habitat: Adults and nymphs are active at night and hide during the day in cracks and crevices, under boards and tree bark. When a blood meal is desired, the host is attacked for only a short time. Larvae may attack day or night.

Identification: Adults are at least 7 mm. long and 5 mm. wide. They are usually reddish-brown, but engorged ticks are slate-blue. Sexual dimorphism is slight. The ticks are flat and leathery, and the integument is wrinkled, bearing many minute setae. There is no shield (scutum).

Distribution and importance: The ticks are mainly found in warm, temperate and semitropic countries. Members of the genus *Argas* are of little economic importance as pests of livestock in the U.S.

Life cycle: Eggs are laid in batches in cracks and crevices of the wall of the chicken house. The hatching period extends 10 days to several months depending on temperature. After hatching, the larvae search for a suitable host, attach, and suck blood about 5 days. After engorgement they drop off, seek a sheltered spot, and molt to become 8-legged nymphs in 4-9 days. Nymphs and adults feed intermittently and are most active at night, hiding in the daytime. Larvae may live 7-8 weeks without food, nymphs about 1 year, and adults 2-3 years.

Transmission: Through contact with infested birds and contaminated premises.

Signs and pathogenicity: In heavy infestations blood loss may result in anemia. The ticks worry the birds at night and interfere with their rest. Egg

production decreases and may even stop. The tick also serves as a vector of
fowl spirochaetosis.

Diagnosis: Ticks may be collected from the birds but usually are readily found
in cracks, crevices, and the bedding of contaminated premises. Plumage becomes ragged, and birds become weak and unthrifty.

Control: These ticks are difficult to control because all stages are highly resistant to acaricides. Control is directed toward destruction or removal of
contaminated debris from the bird's quarters. Carbolineum (anthracene
oil) diluted with kerosene is an effective spray for premises. All litter and
debris must be removed from the building and buried or burned. The spray
should then be applied thoroughly and forced into all cracks, crevices, and
hiding places. Exclude birds from the sprayed facilities until the spray has
soaked in and dried. Malathion and rabon are also effective. Infested birds
may be freed of their ticks by placing them in crates off the ground and allowing the ticks to drop off for 1-10 days. Crates should be sprayed with
an acaricide between batches of birds.

Selected references:

U.S.D.A. 1972. The fowl tick, how to control it. *Leaflet No. 382.*

PARASITE: *Boophilus annulatus* (North American cattle tick, cattle fever tick)

Disease/Infestation: Ixodid acariasis.

Host: Cattle, may also be found on horses and deer.

Habitat: Attached to any part of the body.

Identification: The engorged female is 10-12 mm. long; the male is 3-4 mm.
long. The palpi are very short, and there are no festoons. The spiracular
plate is rounded or oval, and the male has adanal shields.

Distribution and importance: The genus *Boophilus* is considered eradicated
from the U.S. However, it is reintroduced periodically on cattle from
Mexico where the tick is still prevalent. A narrow quarantine zone has
been established along the Texas-Mexico border, and considerable effort,
time, and money are directed toward excluding this pest from the border
area. *Boophilus* is very important as a carrier of cattle tick fever.

Life cycle: *Boophilus* is a 1-host tick. The female completes its parasitic existence on 1 host in an average of 32 days. The female lays about 5,000 eggs
on the ground, and, depending on the season, the eggs incubate 19-202
days. The nonparasitic phase of the life cycle extends 28-288 days. Seed
ticks are very active, climbing on grass or other objects to reach a pass-

ing host. Several generations may be completed annually in a suitable climate.

Transmission: Larvae may be acquired from contaminated grass, weeds, and other plants.

Signs and pathogenicity: With heavy infestations, animals become restless and irritated. To rid themselves of ticks, they rub, lick, bite, and scratch. Irritated areas become raw and may even become secondarily infected. Severe anemia may occur if ticks are numerous. *Boophilus* is of major importance as the sole vector of the agent causing cattle tick fever (see *Babesia bigemina*). The discovery by Smith and Kilborne in 1889-90 that this tick serves as the vector for *Babesia bigemina* was a milestone in the field of parasitology. This was the first demonstration of an arthropod transmitting an infectious disease agent.

Diagnosis: Identification of suspected ticks from the enzootic area or from animals originating near the Texas-Mexico border.

Control: For livestock, tick control is usually practiced on a flock or herd basis. Dairy cattle may be sprayed with such acaricides as arsenic, pyrethrins with synergists, rotenone, or crotoxyphos. Beef cattle may be dipped or sprayed with Delnav, toxaphene, malathion, ronnel, or coumaphos.

Selected references:

Smith, T., and F. L. Kilborne. 1893. Investigations into the nature, causation and prevention of Texas or southern cattle fever. U.S.D.A., *B. A. I. Bulletin No. 1.*
Strickland, R. D., R. R. Gerrish, J. L. Hourrigan, and G. O. Schubert. 1976. Ticks of veterinary importance. A.P.H.I.S., U.S.D.A. *Agr. Handbook No. 485.*

PARASITE: *Cheyletiella parasitivorax*, *C. yasguri* (Rabbit fur mite)

Disease/Infestation: Cheyletid acariasis.

Host: Cat, dog, rabbit, occasionally man.

Habitat: This species is considered by some to be predaceous on parasitic mites. It is found on the fur and the keratin layer of the dermis.

Identification: The female is oval and may be 500 μ long. The palpi are short and stumpy, and the tibial joint is armed with a strong palpal claw curving down.

Distribution and importance: Reported as widely distributed throughout the U.S. These mites appear to be of little economic importance. Infestation of man has been reported but is not of major significance.

Life cycle: Details of the life cycle are not known, apparently completed on 1 host.

Transmission: Direct contact.

Signs and pathogenicity: Although frequently found on healthy animals, the mites may be associated with a dermatosis or mange. Signs associated with this infestation include mild hair loss, scaling, pruritus, serous exudation, and some thickening of the skin.

Diagnosis: Demonstration of mites from dandruff, tufts of hair, or skin scrapings. Mites may be placed in oil or sodium hydroxide for examination.

Control: This mite is quite susceptible to a variety of externally applied acaricides. Rotenone and pyrethrum dusts are recommended for topical treatment of the cat and a benzyl benzoate emulsion for the rabbit. Dogs may be treated by topical application of insecticides such as derris washes, lindane, ronnel, and chlordane. This mite may also be found in litter and bedding, thus pens, cages, kennels, and equipment should be thoroughly cleaned. A suitable spray for kennels and equipment would be chlordane or malathion.

Selected references:

Baker, E. W., T. M. Evans, D. J. Gould, W. B. Hull, and H. L. Keegan. 1956. A manual of parasitic mites of medical or economic importance. Tech. Publ. Natl. Pest Control Assoc., New York.

Ewing, S. A., J. E. Mosier, and T. Foxx. 1967. Occurrence of *Cheyletiella* spp. on dogs with skin lesions. *J. Am. Vet. Med. Assoc.* 151:64-67.

Foxx, T. S., and S. A. Ewing. 1969. Morphologic features, behavior and life history of *Cheyletiella yasguri*. *Am. J. Vet. Res.* 30:269-85.

Maxham, J. W., T. T. Goldfinch, and A. C. G. Heath. 1968. *Cheyletiella parasitivorax* infestation of cats associated with skin lesions of man. *N. Z. Vet. J.* 16:50-52.

PARASITE: *Chorioptes equi, C. bovis, C. caprae, C. ovis* (Foot and tail mange mite, itchy leg mite)

Disease/Infestation: Chorioptic acariasis, leg mange.

Host: Horse, cow, goat, sheep.

Habitat: Found chiefly on the lower part of the hind legs but may spread to the flank and shoulder region. On cattle, mites are frequently found in the tail region, especially in the escutcheon area.

Identification: The mites are ovoid, slightly longer than wide. Unsegmented pedicels with suckers are borne on the 1st, 2nd, and 4th pairs of legs in the female; they are present on all legs of the males. The female may be about 0.4 mm. long.

Distribution and importance: Widely scattered throughout the U.S. This acariasis is not very important economically but may persist for long periods in a herd.

Life cycle: As is true of many mites, details of the life cycle are not fully known.

Transmission: By direct contact. Mites may survive in litter for 3 weeks.

Signs and pathogenicity: Lesions usually are not severe or very conspicuous, and generally the mites do not spread rapidly or extensively. The mites irritate the skin causing serum to exude, and thin crusts and blebs of coagulated serum form on the skin surface. Eventually the skin wrinkles and becomes thickened; itching is not severe. Lesions may diminish during the summer months and then become worse in fall and winter. In horses stamping, biting, and kicking, especially at night, are characteristic signs. The pasterns, especially those of the hind legs, are particularly prone to infestation.

Diagnosis: By identification of the mites from skin scrapings.

Control: Most easily accomplished by sponging the infested areas with a solution of one of the organophosphorus insecticides. An old but effective remedy is the application of warm lime-sulfur wash several times at 10-day intervals.

Selected references:

Sweatman, G. K. 1957. Life history, non-specificity, and revision of the genus *Chorioptes*, a parasitic mite of herbivores. *Can. J. Zool.* 35:641-89.

———. 1958. On the population reduction of chorioptic mange mites on cattle in summer. *Can. J. Zool.* 36:391-97.

PARASITE: *Cnemidocoptes mutans* (scaly-leg mite of chickens), *C. pilae* (scaly-face and scaly-leg mite of parakeets)

Disease/Infestation: Cnemidocoptic acariasis.

Host: Chicken and parakeet.

Habitat: In the chicken, under the epidermal scales of the lower part of the leg or foot. In the parakeet, the mite invades the feather follicles and the epidermis of the face, the foot, and especially the cere.

Identification: Mature forms of these 2 species are very similar morphologically. The body is round and is about 0.4 mm. long. The male is slightly smaller than the female. Both resemble *Sarcoptes scabiei* in shape.

Distribution and importance: Generally distributed throughout North America but infrequently seen in the chicken since the decline of the farm flock. In parakeets the infestation is increasingly important.

Life cycle: Similar to the life cycle of *Sarcoptes scabiei*.

Transmission: Presumably by contact with contaminated bedding, roosts, and equipment.

Signs and pathogenicity: The mites burrow beneath the epidermal scales of the legs and feet causing much irritation, inflammation, and formation of vesicles with a crusty serous exudate. The condition progresses with consequent keratinization, lameness, and distortion and malformation of the foot and lower leg of the bird. In the parakeet the mites invade the epidermis at the base of the cere and the corners of the mouth and adjacent areas. The beak may become distorted and friable. The legs below the hock usually are attacked; hyperkeratosis and sloughing of the keratin may occur.

Diagnosis: Based on typical lesions and the identification of the mite.

Control: In the case of scaly face and leg in the parakeet, a 10% emulsion of benzyl benzoate is applied for 3 days. A 0.2% concentration of lindane in soft paraffin is also claimed effective. Proprietary products such as Dettol, Odylen, and Eurax cream have also been used successfully in treating this infestation.

Selected references:

Blackmore, D. K. 1963. Some observations on *Cnemidocoptes pilae*, together with its effect on the budgerigar. *Vet. Rec.* 75:592-95.

Rickards, D. A. 1975. Cnemidocoptic mange in parakeets. *Vet. Med. Small. Anim. Clin.* 70:729-31.

PARASITE: *Cytodites nudus* (air sac mite)

Disease/Infestation: Cytoditic acariasis.

Host: Chicken, turkey, pheasant, and canary.

Habitat: Respiratory passages and air sacs.

Identification: Adult mites resemble minute, white specks; the female is 500-600 μ long. The dorsal integument is smooth with a few short setae.

Distribution and importance: Appears to be quite widespread but not often reported.

Life cycle: Unknown.

Transmission: Possibly transferred by coughing and sneezing.

Signs and pathogenicity: Small numbers of mites appear to be harmless. Opinions vary concerning the amount of damage caused by the mite. In heavy infestations coughing may result from excess mucus in the trachea and bronchi.

Diagnosis: At necropsy performed soon after death, small white motile specks can be seen on the transparent membranes of the air sacs. To identify mites place them in a drop of water on a slide, apply a cover glass, and examine at 100x magnification.

Control: No attempt has been made to control this pest other than by destruction of infected birds and disinfection of pens.

Selected references:

Baker, E. W., T. M. Evans, D. J. Gould, W. B. Hull, and H. L. Keegan. 1956. A manual of parasitic mites of medical or economic importance. Tech. Publ. Natl. Pest Control Assoc., New York.

Yunker, C. E. 1973. Mites. In *Parasites of laboratory animals*, ed. R. J. Flynn, pp. 425-92. Ames: Iowa State Univ. Press.

PARASITE: *Demodex folliculorum, D. canis, D. equi, D. phylloides, D. bovis, D. ovis,* and *D. caprae* (follicle mite, red mange mite)

Disease/Infestation: Demodectic acariasis.

Host: Dog, man, sheep, goat, horse, cow, pig, and probably many other animals.

Habitat: Hair follicles and sebaceous glands; has also been recovered from lymph nodes and blood.

Identification: Adults are about 250 μ long. Four pairs of short, stumpy legs are grouped at the anterior end of the wormlike, transversely striated body.

Distribution and importance: The species attacking dogs is widely distributed; cattle, sheep, horses, and pigs are less frequently infested.

Life cycle: The life cycle is not well understood. Prenatal infection has been suggested. Various stages of the mite have been observed in the lymph nodes, bloodstream, wall of the digestive tract, spleen, kidney, and urine. The presence of mites in any of these might be accidental. The egg of the mite is spindle shaped. A minute 6-legged larva hatches from the egg; its legs appear as small, stumpy tubercles. The nymph and adult have 8 legs. Little is known of the life cycle or the time necessary for the mite to reach maturity.

Transmission: Generally considered to be by direct contact though, experimentally, it is difficult to transfer this organism from one infected dog to another. The condition of the host seems to be an important factor in susceptibility. Predisposing factors are youth, short hair, malnutrition, poor condition, and debilitation.

Signs and pathogenicity: Two types of infection occur in the dog. In the scaly or squamous form there is usually alopecia and some pruritus, and the thick, wrinkled skin may be reddened, bluish, or copper-colored. In the pustular form of the disease, which is usually preceded by the scaly form, pustules or small abscesses of various sizes may appear on the skin. These lesions are usually invaded secondarily by *Staphylococci*. In typical cases initial signs of the infestation are thickened skin and small hairless patches with reddish pimples and pustules. Lesions are usually seen first around the eyes, muzzle, and forefeet. In neglected cases, the whole body may become involved. Itching in demodectic mange is not as intense as in sarcoptic mange.

Diagnosis: Demonstration of the demodectic mite from a skin scraping. Because animals lick and bite the affected area, mites may be ingested and seen on fecal examination.

Control: Many treatments have been suggested for *D. canis* infestations. Infested animals have been known to recover without treatment; others have shown no improvement in spite of conscientious treatment. Many therapeutic agents have given inconsistent results, and lack of response to established acaricides is not unusual. General control measures consist of good nutrition including a high protein level, clipping and bathing with a mild soap, and the application of an acaricide to affected areas. Rotenone preparations have been widely used as have emulsions of benzyl-benzoate alone or combined with lindane. Ronnel (Ectoral) given orally and in combination with topical applications, has been reported efficacious. An aqueous dip of chlordane has also been widely used. In large animals, suggested treatments have not been very satisfactory. The best results have been attained by incision of the infested nodule and application of tincture of iodine to the lesion. Successful treatment seems related to the thoroughness of application of the acaricide; the material should be worked well into the tissues of the affected areas. If secondary bacterial infection is a problem, antibiotic therapy is indicated.

Selected references:

El-Gindy, H. 1952. The presence of *Demodex canis* in lymphatic glands of dogs. *J. Am. Vet. Med. Assoc.* 121:181-82.

French, F. E. 1964. *Demodex canis* in canine tissues. *Cornell Vet.* 54:271-90.

Greve, J. H., and S. M. Gaafar. 1966. Natural transmission of *Demodex canis* in dogs. *J. Am. Vet. Med. Assoc.* 148:1043-45.

Koutz, F. R. 1954. *Demodex folliculorum* studies. III. A survey of clinical cases in dogs. *J. Am. Vet. Med. Assoc.* 124:131-33.

———. 1955. *Demodex folliculorum* studies. IV. Treatment methods. *North Am. Vet.* 36:129-31, 136.

Kral, F., and R. M. Schwartzman. 1964. Veterinary and comparative dermatology. Philadelphia: Lippincott. Pp. 371-86.

Lucker, J. T., and M. P. Sause. 1952. The occurrence of demodectic mites, *Demodex folliculorum*, in the internal tissues and organs of the dog. *North Am. Vet.* 33:787-96.

Nutting, W. B. 1976. Hair follicle mites (*Demodex* spp.) of medical and veterinary concern. *Cornell Vet.* 66:214-31.

PARASITE: *Dermacentor albipictus* (moose tick, wintertick, horse tick, elk tick)

Disease/Infestation: Ixodid acariasis.

Host: Moose, horse, elk, cattle, and many large wild animals.

Habitat: Tick at all stages may attach anywhere on the body, but usually attaches to the legs, brisket, and along the belly.

Identification: This species is very similar to other *Dermacentor* species. The dorsal shield is marked conspicuously with white and rust. The spiracular plate is oval and contains a few large goblets. The season of collection from the host is an aid to tick identification; *D. albipictus* is found on livestock from autumn until early spring. A long, shaggy hair coat may hide a winter infestation.

Distribution and importance: Widely distributed throughout the northern tier of states. It is found especially in wooded, shrubby, upland country. It was demonstrated experimentally to be a vector of anaplasmosis and is suspected as a carrier of several bacterial pathogens.

Life cycle: This is a 1 host tick. Following copulation the female drops from its host, and the preoviposition period is about 134 days. The female then lays as many as 4000 eggs over a period of 19-42 days and dies. The eggs hatch in 33-71 days. The larvae remain inactive through the summer months and do not search for a host until late fall or early winter. Unfed larvae may live 346 days or more.

Transmission: After hatching, larvae remain clustered to prevent desiccation. They then climb on grass, shrubs, and small trees to await the passing host.

Signs and pathogenicity: Heavy infestations may be associated with loss of appetite, depression, and debilitation. The severe loss of blood caused by heavy infestations may weaken the host, and death may result from debilitation or "tick poverty."

Diagnosis: Collection and identification of the adult tick.

Control: See *D. variabilis.*

Selected references:

Strickland, R. D., R. R. Gerrish, J. L. Hourrigan, and G. O. Schubert. 1976. Ticks of veterinary importance. A.P.H.I.S., U.S.D.A. *Agr. Handbook No. 485.*

PARASITE: *Dermacentor variabilis* (American dog tick, wood tick, dog tick)

Disease/Infestation: Ixodid acariasis.

Host: Dog is the preferred host. Many other mammals, especially small rodents, serve. Meadow mice are commonly infested.

Habitat: Often found around head, neck, and shoulders. *D. variabilis* requires a humid atmosphere and is common in low-brush and grassy areas, especially roadsides and pathways.

Identification: Dorsal shield of male is dark brown with white striping. Unfed ticks are about 6 mm. long, and the engorged female is blue-gray and about 12 mm. long. This tick may be easily confused with *D. venustus* (syn. *D. andersoni*).

Distribution and importance: Widely distributed over the eastern ⅔ of the U.S. and also found in California and Oregon. It is a vector of Rocky Mountain spotted fever, tick paralysis of man and animals, tularemia of rodents, and bovine anaplasmosis.

Life cycle: In the central and northern states adult activity begins in mid-April, reaches a peak in June, and then declines. In southern states ticks in all stages may be found throughout the year. This is a 3-host tick; the life cycle requires 2-3 years. The duration of the life cycle depends on temperture and climate. After attachment, the adult feeds and mates. The female engorges in 5-10 days, detaches, and drops to the ground. An unfed adult female may survive 2-3 years. The preoviposition period is 3-58 days, and egg-laying spans 14-32 days. An egg hatches in 20-57 days. The unfed larva may live 540 days, and the period of larval molt is 6-247 days. The newly emerged nymph may survive 584 days without feeding, and its molting activity takes 24-291 days.

Transmission: Ticks cling to vegetation to await the passing host.

Signs and pathogenicity: May annoy and irritate domestic animals seasonally. Signs are associated with the disease transmitted by the offending tick.

Diagnosis: Identification of the tick.

Control: A small number of ticks may be removed by hand; apply steady traction until each tick relaxes its hold. For small domestic animals washes are more effective than sprays or dusts. Acaricides commonly used are malathion, lindane, Delnav, and rotenone. Dusts recommended are Sevin, lindane, malathion, and rotenone. Dichlorvos-impregnated collars are also useful. Animals quarters may be sprayed with dichlorovos, lindane, or malathion for tick control. In large milk-producing animals no residue of acaricide is allowed. Only minimal residues are permitted in fat of meat-producing stock. For lactating animals arsenic, pyrethrum, rotenone, and crotoxyphos are suggested. For beef cattle and other large domestic animals lindane, Delnav, toxaphene, and malathion are suggested as sprays. Toxaphene, lindane, Delnav, and coumaphos are generally recommended for use as dips. Dips generally provide more complete coverage than sprays. However, spraying is easier, and the equipment is more mobile. If sprays are applied thoroughly, control will be good. If spraying large animals, pressure should be maintained at 200-400 lb. per sq. in. Acaricides may be applied directly to the ear with a squirt-type oil can or a syringe with a few inches of rubber tubing attached to the end.

Selected references:

Cattle tick control. 1976. Wellcome Research Organization, London.

Smith, C. N., M. M. Cole, and H. K. Gouck. 1946. Biology and control of the American dog tick. U.S.D.A. *Tech. Bul. 905.*

Strickland, R. D., R. R. Gerrish, J. L. Hourrigan, and G. O. Schubert. 1976. Ticks of veterinary importance. A.P.H.I.S., U.S.D.A. *Agr. Handbook No. 485.*

PARASITE: *Dermanyssus gallinae* (chicken mite, poultry red mite, roost mite)

Disease/Infestation: Dermanyssid acariasis.

Host: Chicken, wild birds, and man incidentally.

Habitat: Breeds in the bird's environment and usually attacks at night.

Identification: When engorged with blood the adult female is red and is about 1.0 mm. long. Ventral body plates are characteristic. The sternal shield has 2 pairs of setae, the genital plate is truncate, and the anal plate is a broad shield.

Distribution and importance: Widely distributed throughout the U.S. It is an important pest of poultry and can be an annoying pest of man.

Life cycle: The eggs are usually laid after a blood meal. They are deposited in cracks and crevices in the walls of the poultry house or in the nest boxes. Eggs hatch in 2-3 days. The life cycle may be completed in 7-9 days under optimal conditions. Adults may survive 4-5 months without feeding.

Transmission: Accomplished by direct contact with infested birds or contaminated equipment and poultry house litter.

Signs and pathogenicity: Decreased egg production, debilitation, anemia, and, occasionally, death may result from exsanguination. Erythematous papular eruptions may occur on the skin surface. At night birds are frequently uneasy and do not rest well. Birds in production may refuse to lay in infested nests. These mites have been implicated as vectors of St. Louis, western, and eastern equine encephalitis; however, it appears that they do not play an important role in the natural transmission of these diseases.

Diagnosis: Based on identification of the mite. Nymphs and adults feed mostly at night and may be easily collected from the bird at this time.

Control: Because this mite is generally off the host during the day, the cleaning of equipment, cages, and bird's quarters is emphasized rather than treatment of the individual bird. Sevin (carbaryl) controls this mite if applied to houses, perches, and deep litter. It should be applied every 2-3 weeks. Dusts and sprays of malathion are also effective for clearing premises of mites. For treatment of birds and litter, a 4% malathion dust or 0.5% coumaphos dust is effective. Malathion spray has also proved satisfactory. For the treatment of birds only, roosts may be painted with malathion or nicotine sulfate.

Selected references:

Benbrook, E. A. 1965. External parasites of poultry. In *Diseases of Poultry*, ed. H. E. Biester and L. H. Schwarte, pp. 925-64. Ames: Iowa State Univ. Press.

Harrison, J. E., and M. M. Daykin. 1965. The biology and control of ectoparasites of laboratory animals with special reference to poultry parasites. *J. Inst. Animal Techn.* 16:69-73.

U.S.D.A. 1962. Poultry mites: how to control them. *Leaflet No. 383*.

PARASITE: *Laminosioptes cysticola* (flesh or subcutaneous mite)

Disease/Infestation: Laminosioptic acariasis.

Host: Chicken, other domestic and wild birds.

Habitat: Subcutaneous connective tissue of neck, breast, and flank and around vent.

Identification: Adults elongate and may be 260 μ long. The dorsal integument is smooth with few setae. A slight constriction of the body just posterior to the 2nd pair of legs may occur.

Distribution and importance: Widely distributed but of little economic importance.

Life cycle: Unknown.

Transmission: Unknown.

Signs and pathogenicity: Ordinarily these mites appear to have little effect on the bird. They are not markedly pathogenic but may cause the formation of small white nodules several millimeters in diameter. These become calcified after the mites die and have been mistaken for lesions of tuberculosis. Large numbers of these nodules may reduce the market value of birds.

Diagnosis: Accomplished by finding the characteristic nodules and demonstrating the mites or their remains in nodules crushed between glass slides or under a cover glass.

Control: No control is attempted other than the destruction of affected birds.

Selected references:

Baker, E. W., T. M. Evans, D. J. Gould, W. B. Hull, and H. L. Keegan. 1956. A manual of parasitic mites of medical or economic importance. Tech. Publ. Natl. Pest Control Assoc., New York.

Lindquist, W. D., and R. C. Belding. 1949. A report on the subcutaneous or flesh mite of chickens. *Mich. State College Vet.* 10:20-21.

PARASITE: *Latrodectus mactans* (hour-glass spider, black widow spider)

Disease/Infestation: Arachnidism.

Host: Attacks insects, small mammals, and man.

Habitat: Outbuildings, privies, garages, cellars, rodent burrows.

Identification: Glossy, jet-black body with a brick-red, hour-glass mark on the underside of the abdomen. The female may be 3 cm. long including the legs; the male is usually smaller.

Distribution and importance: Widely distributed throughout southern North America.

Life cycle: Development of egg to adult requires about 4 months. Under laboratory conditions the female has lived almost 2 years.

Signs and pathogenicity: This spider is one of the few in the U.S. classed as poisonous. The bite resembles a pinprick. Pain usually develops in the region of the bite and reaches a maximum intensity in 1-3 hours, continuing as long as 48 hours. Signs vary with the individual, but generally, agonizing muscular pain over the abdomen and chest occurs. In addition there may be profuse perspiration, pallor, lowered blood pressure, and dyspnea. In adult humans recovery occurs in 95% of cases.

Diagnosis: History of spider bite and identification of the spider.

Control: Manual destruction of adult spiders and their eggs. Webs and suspected areas should be destroyed and sprayed with an insecticide. A local antiseptic should be applied at the point of injury. Treatment by a physician consists of using a specific antivenom.

Selected references:

Baerg, W. J. 1959. The black widow and five other venomous spiders in the United States. *Univ. Arkansas Expt. Sta. Bul. No. 608.*

Herms, W. B., S. F. Bailey, and B. McIvor. 1935. The black widow spider. *Univ. Cal. Agr. Expt. Sta. Bul. 591.*

PARASITE: *Notoedres cati*

Disease/Infestation: Notoedric acariasis, face and head mange.

Host: Cat, rabbit.

Habitat: Found in burrows in the skin of the ears, face, and front and hind paws. In rabbits the mites may also invade the genital regions.

Identification: The female may be 275 μ long and has suckers on long, unjointed stalks (pedicels) on legs 1 and 2. The male has a sucker on each long, unjointed stalk on legs 1, 2, and 4. The anal opening is distinctly dorsal, an aid in identification.

Distribution and importance: Sparsely scattered throughout North America.

It has been reported as causing considerable trouble in large rabbit colonies.

Life cycle: Similar to that of *Sarcoptes scabiei.*

Transmission: Considered to be by direct contact; infestations are claimed to start at the tip of the ears.

Signs and pathogenicity: The infestation is characterized by persistent pruritus and alopecia. Yellowish encrustations develop on the face and neck, and the skin becomes thickened and wrinkled. If not treated the condition may become generalized. Fatalities have been recorded.

Diagnosis: Identification of the parasite in deep skin scrapings. It must be differentiated from *Sarcoptes*, *Otodectes*, and *Psoroptes.*

Control: The toxicity of chlorinated hydrocarbons and organophosphorus compounds for cats greatly limits the use of these as acaricides. A 3-10% sulfur mixture as an ointment or lotion has been used successfully. Lime-sulfur dip is also satisfactory. For rabbits lime sulfur, lindane, and dimethyl phthalate are recommended.

Selected references:

English, P. B. 1960. Notoedric mange in cats with observations on treatment with malathion. *Aust. Vet. J.* 26:85-88.

Yunker, C. E. 1973. Mites. In *Parasites of laboratory animals*, ed. R. J. Flynn, pp. 425-92. Ames: Iowa State Univ. Press.

PARASITE: *Ornithonyssus sylviarum* (northern feather mite)

Disease/Infestation: Ornithonyssid acariasis.

Host: Domestic fowl, many wild birds, and occasionally man.

Habitat: Usually found on the host but may survive 2-3 weeks off the host. When an infested bird is handled, the mite will quickly crawl over the hands and arms of the examiner. The mite is seen in greatest numbers around the vent, tail, and neck of the bird.

Identification: The adult is about 800 μ long and morphologically is quite similar to the common red mite. A narrow dorsal shield attenuates gradually posteriorly and ends in a blunt point. Identification depends on a critical study of the setation of the dorsal plate.

Distribution and importance: Commonly found on domestic and wild birds throughout the U.S. Heavy infestations are associated with lowered egg production.

Life cycle: The adult spends most of its life on the host. In heavy infestations mites may be found in the host's environment as well. Oviposition occurs on the host, and the life cycle may be completed in about 7 days although more time is usually necessary. The adult may survive 2-3 weeks off a host.

Transmission: By contact with infested birds and use of infested litter.

Signs and pathogenicity: Characteristic signs are soiling of the feathers and thickened, scabby skin particularly in the vent region. Heavy infestations have been credited with causing anemia, decreased weight gain and egg production, and occasionally death. However, the validity of some claims has been questioned. Several viruses, such as those causing Newcastle disease, fowl pox, western equine encephalomyelitis, and St. Louis encephalitis, have been isolated from these mites. It does not appear that this mite plays an important role in the natural transmission of these agents.

Diagnosis: Infestation may be suspected if feathers appear dirty, discolored, and matted, especially in the vent area. Diagnosis is confirmed by collection and identification of the mites.

Control: Involves management of both the birds and their surroundings. Among the older compounds, nicotine sulfate is recommended as a roost paint. A wettable powder spray of coumaphos may be used directly on the birds at the rate of 1 gallon per 100 birds. Malathion dust or spray may be used on roosts, droppings, nests, and litter. Effective and safe control has been accomplished with Sevin dust.

Selected references:

Kraemer, P., and D. P. Furman. 1959. Systematic activity of Sevin in control of *Ornithonyssus sylviarum*. *J. Econ. Entomol.* 52:170-71.

Linkfield, R. L., and W. M. Reid. 1958. Newer acaricides and insecticides in the control of ectoparasites of poultry. *Jour. Econ. Entomol.* 51:188-90.

U.S.D.A. 1964. Poultry mites: how to control them. *Leaflet No. 383.*

PARASITE: *Otobius megnini* (ear tick, spinose ear tick)

Disease/Infestation: Argasid acariasis.

Host: Horse, cattle, sheep, dog, and other wild animals.

Habitat: Larvae and nymphs are usually found in the ears. Fully grown and engorged nymphs drop off the host and seek dry, protected places in cracks and crevices, under logs and fence posts. Here they molt and become adults.

Identification: The adult female is not parasitic. It may be 10 mm. long, is brown, and has a slightly granular integument. The nymph is more or less violin shaped and covering the body are spines that project backward. The male closely resembles the female; neither has a scutum.

Distribution and importance: Original distribution was probably the semiarid or arid areas of the southwestern U.S. However, the current widespread movement of animals over the country has caused an increase in incidence of this pest in many parts of the continent.

Life cycle: Eggs are laid on or near the ground over a period as long as 6 months. They hatch in 18 days or more, and the larvae crawl up vegetation, fence posts and feed bunks to await hosts. Unfed larvae may live off the host for more than 2 months. If they find hosts, they move to the ears, and engorge in 5-10 days. The larvae molt and become nymphs in the ear. Nymphs engorge in about a month, and when ready to molt, they crawl out of the ear onto the ground. There they molt and become adults. The nymphal stages may remain in the ear for 1-7 months. Oviposition may continue as long as 6 months.

Transmission: Usually acquired from a pen, corral, or limited range area where larvae migrate onto host animals.

Signs and pathogenicity: The ticks are a constant and annoying source of irritation. Secondary bacterial infection may produce ulceration of the inner ear causing ear canker. Heavily infested animals appear dull, do not feed well, and lose condition. The ears become highly sensitive; the animal shakes its head constantly and may show signs of deafness. A large amount of blood is lost if many nymphs infest 1 animal.

Diagnosis: Use the otoscope to easily view the ticks within the ear. Using a cotton swab or blunt forceps, the waxy exudate may be removed and examined for larvae and nymphs.

Control: Direct application of 0.5% lindane or toxaphene with a squirt-type oil can or a syringe is a common method of treatment. The tip of the oiler or syringe may be fitted with a short length of rubber tubing to avoid damaging the ear. Ronnel, coumaphos, malathion, and many other acaricidal mixtures have been used with good results.

Selected references:

Strickland, R. D., R. R. Gerrish, J. L. Hourrigan, and G. O. Schubert. 1976. Ticks of veterinary importance. A.P.H.I.S., U.S.D.A. *Agr. Handbook No. 485.*

PARASITE: *Otodectes cynotis* (ear mite)

Disease/Infestation: Otodectic acariasis.

Host: Dog, cat, fox, and ferret.

Habitat: Usually in the external ear.

Identification: A fairly large mite, about 400 μ long. It is easily seen with the unaided eye. The female has tarsal suckers on short, unjointed stalks (pedicels) on legs 1 and 2; leg 4 is quite rudimentary and difficult to see. All 4 pairs of legs in the male bear suckers on short, unjointed pedicels. The anus is terminal.

Distribution and importance: Widely distributed and common, it is an annoying pest of the dog and cat.

Life cycle: The eggs are deposited singly. The life cycle, thought to be similar to that of *Psoroptes* sp., is completed in about 3-4 weeks.

Transmission: Usually by direct contact especially if a bitch is nursing. Transmission from dog to cat may also occur.

Signs and pathogenicity: The mite is usually found deep in the external meatus where it causes intense irritation. This mite is thought to feed on epidermal debris. Infection is frequently bilateral, and the host shakes its head and scratches its ears. Otitis media, with torticollis, circling, and convulsions, sometimes occurs in severe infestations. Auricular hematomas may also develop, and nervous signs similar to those of epileptiform fits may take place. In advanced infestations a purulent inflammation of the external ear may develop. If left untreated, it may lead to a serious infection of the middle and inner ear.

Diagnosis: Mites may be identified by examining the exudate from the ear or by using an otoscope.

Control: The ear should be cleaned and treated with an acaricide. A bland oil or cerumenolytic agent may be introduced into the ear canal, and then the ear may be gently massaged. After cleaning, an acaricide such as 1% rotenone in oil or dimethyl phthalate may be applied every 3rd or 4th day for 4 applications. Benzyl benzoate emulsion also seems effective.

Selected references:

Baker, E. W., T. M. Evans, D. J. Gould, W. B. Hull, and H. L. Keegan. 1956. A manual of parasitic mites of medical or economic importance. Tech. Publ. Natl. Pest Control Assoc., New York.

Camin, J. H., and W. M. Rogoff. 1952. Mites affecting domesticated mammals. *S. Dakota State College Agr. Exp. Sta. Bull.* 10:1-12.

Sweatman, G. K. 1958. Biology of *Otodectes cynotis*, the ear canker mite of carnivores. *Can. J. Zool.* 36:849-62.

PARASITE: *Pneumonyssoides (Pneumonyssus) caninum* (nasal mite of dog)

Disease/Infestation: Nasal acariasis.

Host: Dog.

Habitat: Nasal cavity and paranasal sinuses.

Identification: The oval body is creamy white. The female is 700 μ to 1.5 mm. long. The body cuticle is smooth and bears few setae.

Distribution and importance: Widely distributed throughout the U.S.

Life cycle: Little is known of the life cycle. It has been suggested that the females are ovoviviparous. The nymph stage has not been observed.

Transmission: Method of transmission is unknown but is probably by direct contact.

Signs and pathogenicity: Signs observed are usually a reddening of the nasal mucosae, persistent sneezing, shaking of the head, and rubbing the nose. A marked rhinitis with production of much mucus may be seen.

Diagnosis: The larvae may be seen crawling from the nares of the dog, especially when the host is sleeping. Mites may be recovered on necropsy.

Control: Treatment has not been attempted.

Selected references:

Besch, E. D. 1960. Notes on the morphology of the larva of *Pneumonyssoides caninum. J. Parasitol.* 46:351-54.

Koutz, F. R., D. M. Chamberlain, and C. R. Cole. 1953. *Pneumonyssus caninum* in the nasal cavity and paranasal sinuses. *J. Am. Vet. Med. Assoc.* 122:106-09.

Monlux, W. S. 1940. Mites in nasal passages and sinuses of dogs. *Cornell Vet.* 30:252-55.

PARASITE: *Psorergates ovis* (itch mite of sheep)

Disease/Infestation: Psorergatic acariasis.

Host: Sheep, usually fine-wooled breeds.

Habitat: Found in the superficial layers of the skin, mostly over the withers, sides, or flanks of the host. It is most common in ewes and is seldom seen in sheep younger than 6 months.

Identification: This mite is minute. The female is about 190 μ long, and the male is smaller. The stumpy legs are all about the same size and are almost equally spaced along the sides of the body. The femur of each leg bears a pair of fairly long setae; a large, curved spine is directed inward on the ventral side.

Distribution and importance: Distribution unknown in the U.S. It has been reported from sheep in Ohio and from California and New Mexico.

Life cycle: Little is known of the life cycle of the mite although the developmental stages have been described. The mites live on the surface layers of the skin of fine-wooled breeds.

Transmission: Thought to be by contact or mechanical transfer during shearing.

Signs and pathogenicity: The mites cause a mild skin irritation resulting in occasional biting and scratching. The infestation spreads slowly over the body and becomes generalized in 3-4 years. The wool fibers break easily and the wool is disturbed, disarranged, or pulled out. The skin becomes scaly with dry scabs. Gross lesions are seldom generalized.

Diagnosis: Infestations are extremely difficult to recognize. Shallow skin scrapings should be taken after moistening the skin surface with a drop of mineral oil. To concentrate the mites, the sodium hydroxide maceration and concentration procedure should be used.

Control: The usual acaricides do not seem to be effective in controlling this mite. However, a dip of lime sulfur containing 1% polysulfide of sulfur in addition to a wetting agent is effective if properly applied.

Selected references:

Bell, D. S., W. D. Pounden, B. H. Edgington, and O. G. Bentley. 1952. *Psorergates ovis* — a cause of itchiness in sheep. *J. Am. Vet. Med. Assoc.* 120:117-20.

Davis, J. W. 1954. Studies of the sheep mite, *Psorergates ovis. Am. J. Vet. Res.* 15: 255-57.

Roberts, I. H., and W. P. Meleney. 1965. Psorergatic acariasis in cattle. *J. Am. Vet. Med. Assoc.* 146:17-23.

Roberts, I. H., W. P. Meleney, and H. P. Colbenson. 1965. Psorergatic acariasis on a New Mexico range ewe. *J. Am. Vet. Med. Assoc.* 146:24-29.

PARASITE: *Psoroptes cuniculi* (ear canker mite of rabbit)

Disease/Infestation: Psoroptic otacariasis, ear canker.

Host: Rabbit.

Habitat: Ear and occasionally the head and legs.

Identification: *P. cuniculi* is morphologically indistinguishable from *Psoroptes equi*. The brownish-white female is relatively large, to 750 μ long. The long, jointed pedicels on legs 1, 2, and 4 in the female and on legs 1, 2, and 3 in the male bear suckers. The anus is a simple terminal slit.

Distribution and importance: Widely distributed in laboratory rabbits obtained from most commercial suppliers.

Life cycle: *P. cuniculi* is a nonburrowing mite and feeds on the host by puncturing the epidermis to obtain tissue fluids. The complete life cycle requires about 21 days.

Transmission: By direct contact with infested rabbits.

Signs and pathogenicity: Shaking the head, scratching the ears, hyperemia, and crusts of coagulated serum in the ear canal are characteristic of the infestation. Lesions sometimes occur on the head and legs, and severely infested animals are markedly debilitated. Loss of equilibrium may occur with torticollis.

Diagnosis: Isolation and identification of the mite from the crusty debris inside the ear.

Control: All newly acquired rabbits should be examined and treated. Those showing no signs of infestation should be treated as a precautionary measure. Those showing lesions should be treated weekly until the infestation is eliminated. In severe infestations the brown, crusty exudate must be removed after softening with a few drops of hydrogen peroxide or a mixture of oil and ether. Suitable restraint or even anesthesia is necessary to accomplish this. After cleaning, the ears may be treated with 1 part Canex in 3 parts vegetable or mineral oil. Other effective agents for control of this pest are lindane solution, DDT, and benzyl benzoate emulsion if use is permitted. It may be necessary to treat repeatedly at 1-week to 10-day intervals. Hutches and cages should be thoroughly cleaned and disinfected.

Selected references:

Lund, E. E. 1951. Ear mange in domestic rabbits. *Small Stock Mag.* 35:18-19.
Yunker, C. E. 1973. Mites. In *Parasites of laboratory animals*, ed. R. J. Flynn, pp. 425-92. Ames: Iowa State Univ. Press.

PARASITE: *Psoroptes ovis*, *P. bovis*, and *P. equi* (scab mite)

Disease/Infestation: Scabies, psoroptic acariasis.
Host: Sheep, cattle, horses.
Habitat: Usually the long-wooled or thick-haired areas of the host animal.
Identification: These mites are very host-specific but are morphologically difficult to distinguish. They are oval with suckers on long, jointed pedicels. In the female, suckers are present on long, jointed stalks on legs 1, 2, and 4, and in the male suckers are on the jointed stalks of legs 1, 2, and 3. Adult mites may be 600 μ long.
Distribution and importance: This acariasis has been essentially eradicated from sheep in the U.S. *P. bovis* is occasionally reported from cattle.
Life cycle: The egg is usually laid on the skin surface at the edges of the lesion. It hatches in a few days. The larva feeds, molts, and the pubescent female appears about 5-6 days after hatching. The female usually begins laying eggs about 9 days after hatching from the egg. She lives 30-40 days and lays about 90 eggs.
Transmission: This condition is highly contagious, spreading rapidly from sheep to sheep.
Signs and pathogenicity: The mite punctures the epidermis to obtain lymph, causing an inflammatory swelling that exudes serum. After the serum coagulates and forms a crust, wool is lost. Intense itching causes much scratching and biting resulting in further wool loss. The mite persistently migrates to the undamaged skin at the edge of the lesion. It prefers the heavily wooled parts of the body. As the disease progresses tags of wool are pulled out, and the fleece becomes matted. Finally patches of skin are exposed. In the final stages the skin may become parchmentlike, thickened, and cracked and may bleed. Exercise and activity intensify the itch-

ing. The sheep loses wool by constantly rubbing against fences, posts, farm equipment, or anything else that may serve as a scratching post. Licking the lips and champing the jaws are also characteristic of infested sheep.

Diagnosis: By taking surface scrapings and wool from the edges of active lesions and identifying the mites.

Control: Dip all possibly infected sheep and hand-dress severe lesions and places where the mites may be hiding such as on the scrotum, perineum, sternum, and ears and around the base of the horns. Where use of the chemical is permitted, a dipping with 0.06% lindane will control psoroptic mange in sheep. Toxophene, a 0.5% solution, and lime sulfur are currently approved dips.

Selected references:

Baker, E. W., T. M. Evans, D. J. Gould, W. B. Hull, and H. L. Keegan. 1956. A manual of parasitic mites of medical or economic importance. Tech. Publ. Natl. Pest Control Assoc., New York.

Kemper, H. E. 1952. Sheep scab. *U. S. D. A. Farmer's Bul. 713.*

Kemper, H. E., and H. O. Peterson. 1953. Cattle scab and methods of control and eradication. *U. S. D. A. Farmers Bul. 1017.*

Meleney, W. P., and I. H. Roberts. 1967. Evaluation of acaricidal dips for control of *Psoroptes ovis* on sheep. *J. Am. Vet. Med. Assoc.* 151:725-31.

PARASITE: *Rhipicephalus sanguineus* (brown dog tick)

Disease/Infestation: Ixodid acariasis.

Host: Dog.

Habitat: Skin, often along nape of the neck, on or in the ears, or between the toes. It is seldom found on the cat or man.

Identification: The tick is inornate, with a uniformly reddish-brown scutum. When engorged, it becomes a slaty grey. The basis capitulum has prominent lateral extensions which give the dorsal surface a hexagonal appearance. Stigmal plates are comma shaped, long in the male and short in the female. The male has prominent adanal shields.

Distribution and importance: Widely distributed throughout North America. It is a troublesome pest of dogs and a vector of canine babesiasis as well as other disease agents of man and animals. It is also an annoying household pest.

Life cycle: This 3-host tick feeds almost exclusively on the dog. In warm climates, such as the southern U.S., the life cycle may be completed out-of-doors. In northern areas the life cycle is completed only in houses and heated kennels. The female engorges in 6-50 days; oviposition begins soon after the female leaves the host and continues for 21-29 days. Four to five thousand eggs may be laid under straw and stones, behind baseboard and plaster, and in cracks and crevices in walls. Eggs hatch in about 19 days, and larvae aggregate around the baseboard or at the base of the walls. They may live for 253 days while awaiting a host. Nymphs have been observed to live as long as 183 days. Unfed adults may live as long as 568 days. Under very favorable conditions the life cycle may be completed in 63 days. Such variations in development are due to climatic factors affecting the developmental stages.

Transmission: This pest has rather secretive habits and spends much time under cover. If a dog appears, the tick becomes active and attaches to it.

Signs and pathogenicity: The brown dog tick is fast becoming a serious pest of dogs and a nuisance and embarrassment to those whose residence it may invade. Because the bites are very irritating, the dog suffers much discomfort and blood loss in heavy infestations. This tick is a vector of canine piroplasmosis.

Diagnosis: By identification of the adult. In northern climates finding ticks on the dog, in the home, or in the kennel during late fall and winter is strong evidence of a *Rhipicephalus* infestation.

Control: Control is difficult. In an early infestation manual removal and destruction of ticks may be undertaken. A tick may be removed by applying steady traction until the tick relaxes its hold. A hot match stick or heated knife blade applied to the posterior end of the tick may stimulate it to retract the hypostome and release its hold. After picking off ticks, hands should be thoroughly washed. Rotenone dips and washes are satisfactory acaricides. Chlordane dips and pyrethrum sprays are effective if strains of ticks are not resistant. Kennels should be constructed to minimize hiding places for the ticks. If dwellings are infested, dogs may be housed outside, or these hosts can serve as "bait dogs" to collect ticks. Premises may be sprayed with approved tickicides.

Selected references:

Koutz, F. R. 1941. Identification of ticks. *J. Am. Vet. Med. Assoc.* 97:327.

Strickland, R. D., R. R. Gerrish, J. L. Hourrigan, and G. O. Schubert. 1976. Ticks of veterinary importance. A.P.H.I.S., U.S.D.A. *Agr. Handbook No. 485*.

PARASITE: *Sarcoptes scabiei* var. *canis, suis, equi, bovis* (itch mite, mange mite)

Disease/Infestation: Sarcoptic acariasis, scabies.

Host: Man, domestic and wild mammals. Mites occurring in different species of animals are generally regarded as host varieties.

Habitat: Females are found in tunnels in the epidermis of the skin. Males, larvae, and nymphs may be in the vicinity of the tunnel openings and on the skin surface. Mating occurs on the skin surface or in temporary galleries in the skin. In hogs the neck, shoulders, ears, and withers are usual sites of infestation. In the dog lesions usually appear around the muzzle, eyes, or ears. If not treated, these spread to all parts of the body.

Identification: This minute, greyish-white mite is just visible to the naked eye. The female is 450-500 μ long; the male is about ½ as long. The body of the adult is almost round. The dorsal surface is covered with fine grooves and folds, numerous bristles and spines. The stumpy legs are short, and suckerlike structures are borne at the tips of long, unjointed pedicles on legs 1 and 2 in the female and on legs 1, 2, and 4 in the male. Other legs terminate in bristles. The posterior pairs of legs do not project beyond the border of the body. The larval mite has only 6 legs.

Distribution and importance: Widely distributed throughout North America, most commonly in pigs. This mite is quite important economically.

Life cycle: The gravid female enters the skin and burrows 2-3 mm. in 24 hours. The oval eggs, about 160 μ long, are laid 2-3 at a time as she progresses along the burrow. In 2-3 weeks she deposits 15-20 eggs in the burrow which may be several centimeters long. After she deposits all her eggs, the female usually dies. The egg hatches in 3-8 days, and the 3-legged larva becomes a nymph with 4 pairs of legs. The nymph molts in a pocket in the burrow and either remains there or begins a new tunnel. If female, she molts again and copulates with a wandering male. After copulation she excavates a new tunnel in which her eggs are laid. The entire life cycle requires 2-3 weeks; the adult female's life span in the host is about 1 month.

Transmission: Generally considered to occur by direct contact. Because mites are able to survive off the host for 2-3 weeks, an animal could become infested by contact with contaminated bedding, quarters, or equipment, especially objects used for rubbing and scratching.

Signs and pathogenicity: The sarcoptic mite causes marked pruritus as it tunnels through the skin. Mites found on different species prefer certain locations on their hosts. In general *Sarcoptes* prefers parts of the body sparsely covered with hair such as the rear surface of the udder and scrotum, the neck, and the root of the tail in cattle. In swine lesions are first seen on the head and inside the ears. If the animal is not treated, the entire body surface eventually will become infested. In the dog lesions initially occur on the head but may appear anywhere and may become generalized. Sarcoptic mange lesions are exceedingly aggravating and cause much biting and scratching. Affected areas become inflamed, and serum exudes and dries on the skin surface to form crusts and scabs. Continual rubbing causes large moist or dry scabby areas. As the mites move out into new territory, the vacated areas may dry, and the skin may appear leathery.

Diagnosis: A tentative diagnosis is made on the basis of the signs and lesions and is confirmed by identifying the mites. Examine a deep skin scraping or macerate skin-scraping debris in a 10% solution of sodium or potassium hydroxide. The mites are concentrated and identified from the macerated tissues.

Control: Individual cases of mange may be treated with acaricidal solutions applied by spraying, sponging, or dipping. Dipping is the most thorough and satisfactory means of application for large groups of animals. Lime sulfur may be used if facilities are available for heating the dip to 32-35°C. and if the animals can be held for dipping 4-6 times over a period of 12 days. Lindane or chlordane may be used as a spray or dip where their use is permitted. Small animals may be treated with lime and sulfur. Lindane, chlordane, or benzyl benzoate may be used if permitted. Various organophosphates may also be used either orally or topically. Organophosphate and chlorinated hydrocarbon acaricides are toxic to cats. Rotenone, lime sulfur, and sulfur ointments may be applied to lesions on cats. Premises should be cleaned by spraying with the dip or spray solution used on the infested animals. Pens and kennels should be left unused for 2-3 weeks. Equipment such as blankets, combs, brushes, and harness should also be disinfected and dried thoroughly. A well-balanced, nutritious diet should be available at all times.

Selected references:

Baker, E. W., T. M. Evans, D. J. Gould, W. B. Hull, and H. L. Keegan. 1956. A manual of parasitic mites of medical or economic importance. Tech. Publ. Natl. Pest Control Assoc., New York.

Kral, F., and R. M. Schwartzman. 1964. *Veterinary and comparative dermatology.* Philadelphia: Lippincott. Pp. 343-69.

Sheahan, B. J. 1974. Experimental *Sarcoptes scabiei* infection in pigs: clinical signs and significance of infection. *Vet. Rec.* 94:202-09.

PARASITE: *Trombicula* spp. (chiggers, red bugs, harvest mites)

Disease/Infestation: Trombiculid acariasis.

Host: Cat, dog, chicken, turkey, man, and wild animals.

Habitat: Nymphs and adults are free living, primarily in soil and on vegetation. The larvae, parasites of many species of vertebrates, are of medical and veterinary importance.

Identification: The unengorged larva is reddish and quite small, 200-400 μ

long. The mite feeds on epithelial tissue partially digested by the mite's salivary secretions. These secretions are probably responsible for the severe skin irritation associated with this pest.

Distribution and importance: Widely distributed throughout North America; especially prevalent in the southern part of the continent.

Life cycle: The egg is deposited in soil. After about 10 days the egg hatches, and a 6-legged larva emerges. The larva crawls about the soil surface until a suitable host is found; then it attaches and feeds about 3 days. Then the larva drops from its host to the soil and becomes quiescent. The nymph emerges from the larval skin and feeds. After a rest following feeding, the nymph emerges and then becomes an adult. The life cycle is completed in about 50-55 days. In northern latitudes there are 1-2 generations per year.

Transmission: Contact with larvae crawling on the soil surface and vegetation.

Signs and pathogenicity: Chigger dermatitis is characterized by pustules and wheals that itch intolerably. The larva does not suck blood but injects a digestive fluid that causes cellular disintegration. It is assumed that the digestive fluid causes the "bite" to itch after an hour or so.

Diagnosis: By finding the reddish larvae in scrapings from the site of the lesion.

Control: Several highly effective repellents are available. They may provide short- or long-term protection. Some effective repellents are Deet, dimethyl phthalate, and ethyl hexanediol. Extended protection is obtained by impregnating clothing with a diluted repellent. Insecticidal dusts may be applied to areas such as lawns, campsites, and small recreation areas. Dusts commonly used are 5% chlordane or toxaphene at the rate of 40-50 pounds per acre or a 1% lindane dust at the rate of 50 pounds per acre.

Selected references:

Baker, E. W., T. M. Evans, D. J. Gould, W. B. Hull and H. L. Keegan. 1956. A manual of parasitic mites of medical and economic importance. Tech. Publ. Natl. Pest Control Assoc., New York.

U.S.D.A. 1967. Controlling chiggers. *Home and garden bulletin No. 137.*

Wharton, G. W., and H. S. Fuller. 1952. A manual of chiggers. *Entomological Soc. Wash. Memoir #4.*

B. Insects

PARASITE: *Anopheles*, *Aedes*, and *Culex* spp. (mosquitoes)

Host: Man and many other species of warm-blooded animals.

Habitat: Male mosquitoes are not bloodsuckers. They feed on nectar, plant juices, and other liquids. Female mosquitoes can pierce the skin of many kinds of animals and feed on blood. The female of bloodsucking species normally requires a blood meal before oviposition. Time of feeding is a species characteristic as is place of feeding. Some species feed indoors, and others feed outdoors. Habitats vary from large swampy areas, ponds, and lakes to tree holes, hoof tracks, discarded cans, and water barrels. The natural flight area of an adult is usually less than a mile. However, in a strong wind a mosquito may be carried a long distance.

Identification: Adults, 3-6 mm., are slender and have small spherical heads and long legs. The wing veins, body, head, and legs bear scales. Mosquitoes are usually identified on the basis of wing venation. The long, filamentous antennae have 14-15 segments and are plumose in the males of most species. The adult anopheline mosquito rests and feeds at an angle with the skin surface; the proboscis extends from the mosquito's body in a straight line. The anopheline larva lies flat on the water surface when taking air. In contrast the adult culicine mosquito rests and feeds with the body more or less parallel to the skin surface; the proboscis is directed down perpendicular to the insect body. The culicine larva usually has a long breathing trumpet, and the larva hangs from the water surface at an angle when taking air.

Distribution and importance: Found wherever temperature and moisture are suitable. Some 120 species occur throughout north temperate North America. They are very important as annoying pests of man and animals and as vectors of disease agents for malaria, yellow fever, dengue, filariasis, and eastern and western encephalitis.

Life cycle: All mosquitoes undergo complex metamorphosis. Larvae are commonly known as wrigglers, and pupae as tumblers. Eggs are deposited singly or in rafts on the surface of the water and hatch, releasing larvae after several days incubation. Larvae develop over a period of about 7 days, metamorphose into pupae in 2-3 days, and then hatch as adults. The life cycle is completed in 7-16 days depending on moisture and temperature conditions.

Signs and pathogenicity: Sensitized individuals may react strongly to the injection of mosquito saliva. Considerable swelling may occur at the site of the bite, and marked erythema, pruritus, scratching, and secondary infection may follow. Animals may die, though this is unusual.

Control: Control of adults is attempted by using screens, protective clothing, sprays, nets, and repellents. Organized, large-scale control programs are usually directed toward the larvae. Drainage and application of larvicides are used to control larvae in the breeding habitat. It is difficult to protect stock in the field against the annoyance of mosquitoes.

Selected references:

Bishop, F. C. 1951. Domestic mosquitoes. U. S. D. A. *Leaflet No. 186*: 2-8.

Foote, R. H., and D. R. Cook. 1959. Mosquitoes of medical importance. U. S. D. A. *Agr. Handbook No. 152.*

Horsfall, W. R. 1955. Mosquitoes, their bionomics and relation to disease. New York: Ronald Press.

PARASITE: *Bovicola bovis*, *B. equi*, *B. ovis*, and *B. caprae* (chewing louse of large animals, biting louse, red louse)

Disease/Infestation: Phthirapterosis.

Host: Cattle, horses, sheep, and goats.

Habitat: Epidermal surface especially of the neck, withers, and around the root of the tail.

Identification: Small, 1-2 mm. long. These dorso-ventrally flattened, wingless insects have 3 pairs of legs and broad, flat heads with mandibles adapted for chewing. They are host-specific to a remarkable extent, and usually not more than 1 species of chewing louse is found on any mammalian species.

Distribution and importance: Generally throughout North America. Lousiness is a serious economic condition in many localities.

Life cycle: The life cycle is completed in 3-4 weeks. The egg hatches in 5-7 days, and the young louse matures in 15-18 days. If separated from the host, the adult may live 7 days; an egg separated from the host may hatch in 2-3 weeks in warm weather.

Transmission: Usually by direct contact; may also be spread by contaminated curry combs, brushes, blankets, and other equipment.

Signs and pathogenicity: Skin irritation and pruritus resulting in much scratching, itching, licking, and biting of infested areas. General unthriftiness, rough hair coat, and loss of weight or lowered milk production are usually evident. Animals inadequately or poorly fed, overcrowded, and/or subject to unsanitary conditions are often infested. Individual animals differ in their susceptibility to various species of lice. Some animals in a herd may have few lice while others in the same herd are severely infested.

Diagnosis: Demonstration of nits and lice in hair clippings or collection of lice by using a comb. Lice may be easily overlooked in animals in the northern U.S. where the cold climate stimulates growth of a very heavy hair coat.

Control: Several highly effective insecticides, if properly applied, will control lice. These may be sprays, dips, powders, dusts, or systemic insecticides, and they may be poured on, injected, sprayed, or applied by hand, dust gun, or back rubber. Dusts usually are not effective in eradicating lice, but they will hold the population in check. When the weather is unsuitable for spraying or dipping in cold climates, a dust must be used. The use of insecticides on dairy cattle is highly restricted, but many first-class insecticides are available for use on beef animals. Spraying or dipping must be thorough for good results. Usually 2 treatments about 14 days apart are necessary for eradication of lice. Restrictions on the use of insecticides, tissue residue tolerances, and minimum drug withdrawal times are constantly revised. It is essential that the veterinarian is well informed of both state and federal restrictions on the use of pesticides.

Selected references:

Kingscote, A. A., J. K. McGregor, and D. J. Campbell. 1956. Cattle lice and how to control them. *Ont. Dept. Agr. Bul. No. 517.* Pp. 3-15.

Matthysse, J. G. 1946. Cattle lice, their biology and control. *Agr. Expt. Sta., Cornell Univ. Bull.* 832:3-67.

PARASITE: *Cimex lectularius* (bedbug, wall louse, mahogany flat)

Disease/Infestation: Cimicidosis.

Host: Small laboratory animals, birds, and man.

Habitat: These bugs feed nocturnally, hiding in cracks and crevices during the day. At night they often travel considerable distances to find hosts.

Identification: About 4-5 mm. long. The yellow to reddish-brown adult is oval and dorso-ventrally flattened. The bedbug has a conspicuous pair of long, 4-jointed antennae, 2 large compound eyes, and a body covered with spinose bristles and hairs. The adult has a pair of ventral, thoracic, stink glands.

Distribution and importance: Widespread throughout temperate North America but no longer a pest of major importance. It is sometimes a serious pest in animal colonies, pigeon lofts, and poultry houses.

Life cycle: The female bug deposits creamy-white eggs in batches of 10-50, and the young hatch in about 10 days. Under suitable conditions of temperature and humidity, the young mature 8-13 weeks after hatching. All stages can endure prolonged starvation, and adults have been kept alive for 1 year without food.

Transmission: This pest is commonly dispersed in public conveyances and meeting places. The insects are easily carried in clothing or luggage and may even be distributed with secondhand furniture and bedding.

Signs and pathogenicity: Welts and local inflammation constitute an allergic reaction to the saliva of the bug. The bedbug does not appear to do much harm except that it is exceedingly annoying.

Diagnosis: By finding the living insects, their eggs, or cast skins. Characteristic "bug marks" may be seen on walls and decorated areas. Some people can recognize a characteristic bedbug odor in infested areas.

Control: Because this pest does not fly, contact residual insecticides work well after thorough cleaning of the premises. Chlordane and malathion are highly effective.

Selected references:

U.S.D.A. 1959. How to control bed bugs. *Leaflet No. 453.* Pp. 2-7.

Usinger, R. L. 1966. *Monograph of Cimicidae (Hemiptera-Heteroptera). No. 7.* College Park, Maryland: Thomas Say Foundation.

PARASITE: *Cochliomyia hominivorax* (Syn. *Callitroga hominivorax*) (screwworm)

Disease/Infestation: Obligatory myiasis.

Host: Any living warm-blooded animal.

Habitat: Living tissue and fresh lesions.

Identification: Adult fly is 10-15 mm. long. The body is metallic blue, and the face is reddish-orange. The dorsal surface of the thorax has 3 dark stripes. The mature larva is about 12 mm. long with distinct bands of spines around each body segment. The larva has a pair of tracheae extending from the posterior spiracles forward into the body cavity. The tracheae are deeply pigmented for about $1/3$ their length.

Distribution and importance: Formerly a very important insect pest of livestock in the southern U.S. Annual losses were 50-100 million dollars until the eradication program was completed. Geographical distribution may be extended if infected animals are transported by truck, railroad, or possibly by plane.

Life cycle: The female lays several thousand eggs in batches on living flesh of warm-blooded animals. The egg usually hatches in about 24 hours, and the larva matures in 4-7 days. Duration of pupation, usually about 1 week, varies with temperature. The fly commonly overwinters in the pupal stage. Completion of the life cycle requires about 21 days.

Transmission: Direct contact with the adult fly.

Signs and pathogenicity: Screwworms feed as a group, burrowing deeply into *fresh* tissue. Small inconspicuous fresh wounds not only attract screwworms, but as the tissues decompose, blowflies and houseflies are attracted by the wound exudate. Infected animals characteristically isolate themselves from the herd and seek protection in shade and bushes. The screwworm larvae penetrate fresh tissue which they liquidize. The necrotic tissue becomes foul, and if the animal is not treated death often follows.

Diagnosis: Identification of adult flies or larvae is not easy; confirmation of identification by a specialist is highly desirable.

Control: Based on avoiding wounds during the fly season, inspecting animals frequently, and treating infestations to kill the larvae. Breeding should be planned so that young are not born at the peak of the fly season. Castration, dehorning, docking, and branding should be done in cool weather. Fly and tick control should be practiced.

In the late 1950s, the U.S.D.A. launched a program of eradication of screwworm from the southern U.S. The female screwworm fly mates only once; therefore, if she mates with a sterile male, she does not reproduce. The biological control program is based on these features of the life cycle. Screwworm larvae can be reared on artificial media, and just before emergence the pupae are exposed to gamma irradiation sufficient to cause sexual sterility but no other impairment of the pupa. Sterile flies are distributed over the area of infestation by plane. Females native to the area mate with the liberated sterile males and do not reproduce. Eventually native males are outnumbered by sterile males and no eggs are fertilized. Thus native flies are eliminated. The eradication program has been extended throughout the southern U.S., and presently enough sterile flies are distributed along both sides of the Mexico-U.S. border to significantly decrease migration northward. Complete elimination of screwworm from the U.S. by this procedure probably will not be accomplished until the fly is eradicated from Mexico. For control of herd or individual infestations, mixtures like E.Q. 335 are highly effective as are sprays and dusts of coumaphos and ronnel.

Selected references

Baumhover, A. H., A. J. Graham, B. A. Bitter, D. E. Hopkins, W. D. New, F. H. Dudley, and R. C. Bushland. 1955. Screw-worm control through release of sterilized flies. *J. Econ. Entomol.* 48:462-66.

Laake, E. W. 1936. Economic studies of screwworm flies, *Cochliomyia* species with special reference to the prevention of myiasis of domestic animals. *Iowa State College J. Sci.* 10:345-59.

PARASITE: *Cuterebra* spp. (rodent bot fly, rabbit bot, or warble)

Disease/Infestation: Cutaneous myiasis.

Host: Cats, dogs, wild rodents and lagomorphs.

Habitat: In cystlike lesions in subcutaneous connective tissue.

Identification: The beelike adult fly is large, about 20 mm. long, and is a shiny black or blue. It is not parasitic and is seldom seen. The mature larva, about 25 mm. long, is coal-black and is covered with many stout, cuticular spines.

Distribution and importance: Distributed throughout North America; not a pest of major importance but of concern to the pet owner and small animal practitioner.

Life cycle: The adult female lays eggs near the entrance of a rodent burrow. The egg hatches, and the larva penetrates the skin of the host producing a large subcutaneous cyst. In about a month the larva matures and drops from the host to pupate. The fly apparently overwinters as a pupa. On emergence of the adult fly the following spring, mating occurs, and the female is on the wing only for about 2 weeks.

Transmission: It is thought that the hatched larva penetrates the skin around the mouth and nose. After entry larvae migrate to various locations.

Signs and pathogenicity: A subcutaneous abscesslike cyst containing the larva develops. In puppies and kittens the larvae are frequently found in the submandibular region. In rodents a parasitic orchitis may be caused by those species whose habitat is the scrotum.

Diagnosis: Identification of the larva removed from the abscesslike cyst.

Control: Removal of the larva by surgical enlargement of the abscess and careful extraction of the grub. Rupture of the larva may result in anaphylaxis. Screened cages and hutches may be used to keep out adult flies.

Selected references:

Dalmat, H. J. 1943. A contribution to the knowledge of the rodent warble flies (*Cuterebridae*). *J. Parasitol.* 29:311-18.

Sillman, E. 1956. Further laboratory and field observations on the ecology of some Ontario Cuterebridae (Diptera), in particular, *Cuterebra angustifrons* Dalmat 1942. *Ann. Rept. Ent. Soc. Ont.* 87:28-40.

PARASITE: *Eristalis tenax* (adult: drone or hover fly; larva: rat-tailed maggot)

Disease/Infestation: Pseudomyiasis.

Host: Nonparasitic, associated with host's habitat.

Habitat: Adult flies, found near flowers, feed on nectar and pollen. Larvae, found in polluted water, feed on decaying vegetation.

Identification: The adults resemble large honey or drone bees. They have strong bodies, 15-38 mm. long. The larvae are known as rat-tailed maggots because the breathing tubes look like long tails.

Distribution and importance: Widely distributed throughout North America. It is important only because the owner is concerned when larvae are observed in the gutter behind cattle in the barn.

Life cycle: Eggs are deposited in water polluted with excrement or decaying vegetation. The rat-tailed larvae hatch and later, pupate.

Transmission: Eggs are occasionally deposited close to the vulva, and larvae may migrate into the vagina. Larvae may be ingested with water contaminated with feces, urine, or effluent from cesspools or privies.

Signs and pathogenicity: No clinical signs are associated with this fly at any stage.

Diagnosis: Identification of rat-tailed larvae.

Control: None indicated other than collection and destruction of larvae.

PARASITE: *Gasterophilus intestinalis* (common horse bot), *G. nasalis* (chin- and throat-bot fly), *G. hemorrhoidalis* (nose bot fly)

Disease/Infestation: Gastric myiasis.

Host: Horse, mule, and occasionally man.

Habitat: Adults are on the wing from June until the first autumn frost. The adult lives 1-2 weeks. The female hovers close to the horse and darts in cementing each egg to the end of a hair. The larvae of all 3 species spend about a month in the mouth and then migrate to the stomach and attach to the mucosa there. The red larvae of *G. intestinalis* eventually colonize the cardiac portion of the stomach, rarely the fundic or pyloric areas. The pale yellow larvae of *G. nasalis* attach in the region of the pylorus and in the duodenum. The reddish larvae of *G. hemorrhoidalis* are usually in or

near the pyloric region. Before final passage to the outside, the larvae of
this species reattach on the mucosa of the rectum for a few days.

Identification: The brown adult fly, 13-18 mm. long, is hairy and beelike
with 1 pair of wings. The 3rd-stage larva can be identified by the spine pattern. A single row of spines is present on each segment of the larva of *G.
nasalis*. In *G. intestinalis* and *G. hemorrhoidalis* each larval segment bears
2 rows of spines. In *G. intestinalis* spines on the 1st row are larger than
those on the 2nd row. In *G. hemorrhoidalis* the spines on the 1st row are
smaller than those on the 2nd row.

Distribution and importance: Generally found throughout North America. *G.
nasalis* appears to be most common in the Rocky Mountain region of the
country. During oviposition adult flies annoy horses, which may run away
or become unmanageable. The adult fly does not bite or sting. Opinions
vary greatly concerning the harmful effects of the larvae in the stomach.

Life cycle: Eggs of these 3 species vary in color and in the areas where they
are laid. Those of *G. intestinalis* are glued to hairs on almost any part of
the body but especially to the hairs of the forelegs and shoulders. They
hatch in about 7 days if subjected to moisture and friction, which are provided by the host licking, rubbing, and slobbering over its lower front legs.
The eggs of *G. hemorrhoidalis* are attached to the hairs around the lips; the
larvae emerge in 2-3 days without stimulation and crawl into the mouth,
penetrating the tissues. *G. nasalis* lays eggs on hairs in the submaxillary region, and they hatch in about a week without stimulation. Following pupation for 1-2 months, the adult fly emerges and copulates. Egg-laying begins in early summer. The entire life cycle is completed in about 1 year.

Signs and pathogenicity: In most animals, bots do not produce any signs of
disease especially if the host is well nourished. A nonspecific digestive disturbance may occur. The major economic losses are usually associated
with the activity of the adult fly. The opinions regarding the importance
of bots in horses are quite variable. However, a massive larval infection
causes gastric ulceration and mechanical interference that would have
an unfavorable effect on the host.

Diagnosis: The eggs may be identified by color, mode of attachment to the
hair, and site where deposited. The eggs of *G. hemorrhoidalis* are black;
those of the other species are pale yellow. Larvae may be identified by
size and arrangement of the spines.

Control: Animals should be groomed frequently. Clipping will remove the
eggs but is not always popular among owners. The eggs may be hatched by
washing or sponging the infested area with water at 40-43°C. After hatching, the larvae can be washed onto the ground to die. Shade or darkened

shelters that animals can enter during times of fly activity are claimed to give some relief because flies usually avoid shady areas. Horses should be treated in fall about 1 month after the first killing frost has destroyed all flies. Piperazine carbon bisulfide complex has been effective and widely used. Recently dichlorvos and trichlorfon have been widely used.

Selected references:

Dove, W. E. 1918. Some biological and control studies of *Gasterophilus haemorrhoidalis* and other bots of horses. *U. S. D. A. Bul. No. 597.*

Drudge, J. H., E. T. Lyons, and S. C. Tolliver. 1975. Activity of organophosphorus compounds against oral stages of *Gasterophilus intestinalis* and *Gasterophilus nasalis. Am. J. Vet. Res.* 36:251-53.

U.S.D.A. 1973. Horse bots—how to control them. *Leaflet No. 450.*

PARASITE: *Haematobia irritans* (Syn. *Siphona irritans*) (horn fly, Texas fly)

Disease/Infestation: Dipterosis.

Host: Cattle.

Habitat: Spends most of its adult life on cattle. It feeds and rests on the animal between feedings, leaving the host only to oviposit on fresh cow manure. Adults usually rest on the topline of the animal or over the withers, or they cluster in hundreds around the base of the horn.

Identification: On casual examination, it is very similar to the stable fly but about half as large; the horn fly is 3-4 mm. long.

Distribution and importance: Widespread throughout U.S.; probably causes greater losses in livestock production than any other bloodsucking fly.

Life cycle: The eggs are almost always deposited in groups of 5 or 6 on the side of a cake of fresh cow manure or on the grass or soil beneath it. About 20 eggs are deposited at a time, but each female can lay 400 eggs in her lifetime. In warm weather the egg hatches in 24 hours, and the larva reaches maturity in 4-8 days. It pupates and hatches in 6-8 days. In hot, humid weather the life cycle can be completed in 10-14 days.

Transmission: The adults do not fly much. They move from place to place by staying on the host.

Signs and pathogenicity: Harmful effects of the hornfly are chiefly irritation and annoyance which cause disturbed feeding, improper digestion, loss of flesh, and reduction in milk yield. Milk production may be reduced 10-20% at the height of the fly season. Populations of 10,000 flies per animal have been observed; such a population would cause very severe blood loss each day.

Diagnosis: The fly usually feeds with the head toward the ground. The small size of the fly and the long periods it spends resting on the host are characteristic features.

Control: Because this fly lives almost continuously on the same host, the opportunity for control is excellent. On beef cattle, high-pressure spraying every 2-3 weeks with carbaryl, malathion, toxaphane, coumaphos, or ronnel is highly effective. For dairy cattle, dichlorvos, crotoxyphos, coumaphos, and pyrethrum may be used. Back rubbers impregnated with appropriate insecticides may be used on dairy and beef cattle. Dusting and self-dusting bags also control horn flies. Great care must be taken to prevent contamination of milk or milking equipment. Some natural control is possible by running hogs with cattle. Cattle droppings are thereby dispersed and dried.

Selected references:

Bruce, W. G. 1964. The history and biology of the horn fly, *Haematobia irritans* (Linnaeus); with comments on control. *N. C. Agr. Expt. Sta. Tech. Bul. 157.*
McLintock, J., and K. R. Depner. 1954. A review of the life history and habits of the horn fly, *Siphona irritans* (L.) (Diptera, Muscidae). *Can. Entomol.* 86:20-33.

PARASITE: *Haematopinus asini* (sucking louse of horse), *H. suis* (hog louse), *H. eurysternus* (short-nosed cattle louse), *Linognathus pedalis* (foot louse of sheep), *L. vituli* (long-nosed or blue louse of cattle), *Solenopotes capillatus* (hairy cattle louse)

Disease/Infestation: Phthirapterosis.

Hosts: Horse, pig, cattle, and sheep.

Habitat: Usually found on somewhat protected areas of the host. Preferred areas are the side of the neck, brisket, back, between the legs, and around the muzzle, cheek, ears, and eyes.

Identification: *L. vituli* is about 2.5 mm. long and has a long, narrow head and slender body. *H. eurysternus* is about 3.5 mm. long and is broader than *L. vituli*. *S. capillatus* is smaller; it may be 1.5 mm. long. The eggs of these 3 species are quite similar. *H. suis* is the only louse found on the pig.

Distribution and importance: Most species occur throughout North America.

Life cycle: Considerable variation among species but the life cycle is generally as follows. Eggs are laid for 10-15 days and hatch after about 14 days. Nymphs mature in 15-18 days. Under optimal conditions the life cycle may be completed in about 1 month.

Transmission: Usually occurs through direct contact with an infested host.

Signs and pathogenicity: Infested cattle suffer continual worry and irritation. A sucking-louse infestation may produce severe illness, though in adults it usually produces lowered vitality, general unthrifty condition, anorexia, loss of hair, and in some cases, severe anemia. Severely infested calves with tender skin may show signs of colic and may die.

Diagnosis: By demonstration of lice from the skin and nits attached to the hairs.

Control: Apply insecticide directly to the skin as a dust, dip, spray, or a systemic insecticide. There are strict limits on the insecticides that may be applied to dairy cattle and milking goats. In winter, hand dusting, dust bags, and back-rubbing devices are all valuable aids in louse control. Spraying and dipping are widely practiced, and usually 2 fall treatments about 14 days apart will eradicate an infestation. Dipping is usually more dependable than spraying, though spraying is effective if done thoroughly. Housing and yards should be cleaned and left vacant for at least 20 days depending on air temperature and relative humidity.

Selected references:

Matthysse, J. G. 1946. Cattle lice: their biology and control. *Cornell Univ. Agr. Expt. Sta. Bul. No. 832.*

PARASITE: *Hypoderma lineatum*, *H. bovis* (larvae called cattle grubs or ox warbles and adults called heel or bomb flies)

Disease/Infestation: Cutaneous myiasis.

Host: Cattle, occasionally horses, and rarely man.

Habitat: The adult fly, common in midsummer, is active on warm days. Cattle are annoyed when the female fly attaches eggs to the hairs on the legs and sometimes the body. *H. bovis* lays its eggs singly; *H. lineatum* deposits them in a row of 6 or more eggs per hair. The fly is very persistent in approaching the host, and a female may deposit 100 or more eggs on 1 individual. In early spring the larva appears in the subcutaneous tissues of the back. During early summer it falls to the ground, pupates, and ultimately emerges as an adult fly.

Identification: Adult flies are hairy and approximately the size of honeybees. *H. bovis* is about 15 mm. long and *H. lineatum* about 13 mm. Adults have no functional mouthparts. The thorax of *H. bovis* is densely covered with yellow hairs anteriorly and black hairs posteriorly; the terminal hairs of the abdomen are yellow. *H. lineatum* has a fairly uniform hairy covering of mixed brownish-black and white with some red-orange hairs on the terminal segment of the abdomen. The young larva is almost white, changing to yellow and then to dark brown as it matures. The full-grown larva of *H. bovis* is about 28 mm. long, that of *H. lineatum* about 25 mm. In both species each larval segment bears flat tubercles. Small spines are present on all segments but the last in *H. lineatum* and on all but the last 2 in *H. bovis.*

Distribution and importance: *H. lineatum* is widely distributed throughout North America; *H. bovis* is usually found in the northern regions of the continent. Major economic losses are associated with weight loss, decrease in milk yield, traumatic injury resulting from fright, and damages to hides from grub perforation.

Life cycle: The life cycles of the species are similar. The duration of a particular stage varies considerably with the weather and may be correlated with regional climatic conditions. The hairy, beelike adults fly rapidly and deposit the white eggs, each about 1 mm. long, on the hairs of the legs and the lower abdominal region. The eggs hatch in 2-6 days, and the larvae burrow into the host's tissues. For several months they travel through connective tissues. The larvae secrete proteolytic enzymes that dissolve the tissues and provide nourishment. *H. lineatum* larvae aggregate for 2-4 months in the submucosa of the esophagus, whereas *H. bovis* larvae migrate along nerve tissue and aggregate in the epidural fat of the spinal canal. The larva is then about 15 mm. long and begins its final migration through the connective tissue, eventually arriving in the subdermal tissues of the back. After 40-60 days development in the back, the mature larva emerges through the breathing hole, falls to the ground, and pupates. It is then about 25 mm. long and 8 mm. or more in diameter. Depending on weather, the adult emerges in 1-3 months. On hatching, the adults copulate and for about 1 week annoy and terrorize cattle. The adults do not feed or bite, and they die after a week of hectic activity.

Transmission: Adult flies attack hosts intermittently to lay eggs.

Signs and pathogenicity: The approach of the flies frightens cattle, and they attempt to escape by running to shade or into water. Significant decreases in milk yield and body weight may occur during the summer months. Cattle may injure themselves running wildly to avoid fly attack. The activity of 1 fly laying eggs on the lower leg is sufficient to stampede a herd of grazing cattle. Connective tissue around the migrating and growing larvae becomes irritated, and the adjacent tissue becomes greenish-yellow and must be trimmed and discarded when the cattle are butchered. Anaphylactic reactions also may occur in sensitized animals if larvae die in situ or are crushed during manual extraction.

Diagnosis: Finding eggs on the hair of animals and observing the larvae under the skin of the back.

Control: Larvae may be removed mechanically from docile, thin-skinned animals, or the lesions on the back may be treated with a larvicide. Rotenone, the active principle of the derris root, has been widely used as a larvicide. The treatment is highly effective, but for good control repeated treatments are necessary. Unfortunately the larvae are killed only after the journey through the tissues and the damage to flesh and hide are complete. The organophosphorus systemic insecticides have been highly effective in controlling larvae in the early stages of migration. The insecticide is absorbed by the host and kills the migrating grubs in all parts of the body before they reach the back of the host. Effective grub control can be accomplished with these systemic chemicals; however, certain precautions must be taken. Cattle should be treated as soon as the adult fly season is over, usually about 1 month after the first frost. They should not be treated later than 8-12 weeks before the anticipated appearance of grubs in the back. Migrating *H. lineatum* larvae aggregate in large numbers at this time in the submucosal tissues of the esophagus. If larvae are rapidly killed by systemic insecticides, a massive, transitory inflammatory reaction may occur. Swelling may completely occlude the esophageal lumen, and swallowing and eructation may be impaired. In severe cases, the affected animal may die of bloat if not treated. Migrating larvae of *H. bovis* may also be in the epidural fat at this time, and if rapidly killed with systemic insecticides, a transitory irritation of spinal tissue and paralysis may result. Pour-on, spray, and feed-additive formulations are readily available. Pour-on agents suggested are coumaphos, famophos, ruelene, and trichlorfon. Sprays used are ruelene, coumaphos, and trichlorfon. Famophos and ronnel have been used as feed additives. No systemic insecticide should be supplemented or used in combination with another because the actions may be synergistic and highly toxic. These additives must not be fed to lactating animals.

Selected references:

Scharff, D. K. 1950. Cattle grubs – their biologies, their distribution and experiments in their control. *Montana State College, Agr. Expt. Stat. Bul. No. 471.*

Schwartz, W. L., F. C. Faries, J. F. Buxton, and L. P. Jones. 1974. Sudden death of a bull with oesophageal infestation of *Hypoderma* larvae. *Southwestern Vet.*:188-90.

U.S.D.A. 1970. How to control cattle grubs. *Leaflet No. 527.*

PARASITE: *Melophagus ovinus* (sheep ked, sheep tick)

Disease/Infestation: Melophagiasis.

Host: Sheep.

Habitat: Found on coarse- and medium-wooled breeds of sheep. The larva is attached to a wool fiber by the female and almost immediately transforms into a pupa. The adult lives among the wool fibers and on the skin of various parts of the body but is most common in the region of the neck, shoulders, and belly.

Identification: This pest is a true insect, a wingless, hairy fly about 4-6 mm. long. The head, thorax, and abdomen are readily delineated. The brown adult has 6 legs, and the feet bear vicious-looking claws.

Distribution and importance: Found in most parts of the U.S. where sheep are raised. Keds are responsible for considerable economic loss because poor condition results from host irritation and annoyance. The sheep's skin is pierced by the ked as it obtains blood and lymph. A permanent, pimplelike lesion known as cockle results. Efforts to relieve irritation by biting, scratching, and rubbing of the lesions may seriously damage the fleece.

Life cycle: The female ked retains the egg in which a larva develops in about 7 days. When laid the larva is covered by a soft membrane which turns brown and becomes a hard shell surrounding a pupa in a few hours. The pupa is cemented to wool fiber, and a young ked emerges after about 20 days, matures, and copulates. The adult ked may live 3-4 months, and during this period a female produces 10-12 larvae. A satiated female may live apart from the host about 1 week to 10 days. Most larvae are produced in winter and spring; fewer are produced during summer.

Transmission: Keds are usually acquired by contact with infested sheep.

Signs and pathogenicity: Keds consume a significant quantity of blood and cause intense itching and skin irritation. Infested sheep rub, bite, and scratch themselves, pulling out wool and breaking wool fibers. Ked feces dirty and discolor the wool with stains that are difficult to wash out. Infested flocks do not eat well, and losses result because growth is slow. The skin of young lambs is especially sensitive to the ked bites. In severe infestations the animals may show some anemia.

Diagnosis: Identification of the adult and pupa and the general appearance of the fleece.

Control: Spring shearing markedly reduces the population of pupae and adult keds. Sheep are usually treated after shearing to ensure a thorough job whatever procedure is employed. At least 10 days should elapse between shearing and treatment to allow healing of all shear-cuts. If vats are available, dipping is the most effective method of treatment. However, spraying is preferred by many owners because it is faster, more mobile, easier, and safer than dipping. If dipping is selected, each animal must be in the dip for at least 1 minute, and the head should be submerged twice for a few moments. Lambs too young to be dipped in the regular tank should be hand dipped in a wash tub or barrel. All sheep should be piloted through the dipping vat and carefully watched during the process. A wide variety of highly effective insecticides is available for use as dips, sprays, or dusts. Some currently recommended are coumaphos, malathion, methoxychlor, and ronnel. For small flocks of short-wooled breeds, low pressure sprayers operating at 100-200 pounds per square inch are satisfactory. For breeds with heavy fleece or for range animals 200-400 pounds per square inch is more effective.

Selected references:
U.S.D.A. 1953. The sheep tick and its eradication. *Farmers Bul. No. 2057.*

PARASITE: *Musca autumnalis* (face fly)

Disease/Infestation: Dipterosis.
Host: Cattle, horses.
Habitat: Around eyes, nostrils, and muzzle.
Identification: Morphologically very similar to the housefly. It is a little larger than the housefly and can be differentiated by the specialist on the basis of the proximity and angle of the interior margins of the eyes and of distinctive abdominal coloration of the male and female. The larva is yellowish, and the pupa is dirty white.
Distribution and importance: First observed in the northeastern U.S. in 1952. It has spread from coast to coast and is prevalent throughout the country except in the southern-most regions. This fly is very annoying, causing reduced milk production and weight gain.
Life cycle: Similar in most respects to that of the housefly. The eggs are deposited in fresh cow feces, and the life cycle is completed in about 14 days. Adults that have not mated hibernate in houses and barns and may be a nuisance. The female feeds on secretions around the head; males are seldom found on animals and usually rest on fence posts, barn doors, and tree leaves. Both sexes spend the night on vegetation, not on the animal. They do not follow animals into the barn.
Transmission: During the daytime they fly from one host to another.
Signs and pathogenicity: Like the housefly, the face fly is important because it annoys and irritates livestock. Cattle often form groups with their heads together in the center. The habits and structure of the face fly are well suited to the transmission of the pathogen associated with infectious bovine keratitis (pink eye).
Diagnosis: A tentative diagnosis may be based on observing these flies concentrated around the eyes and nostrils of cattle. A definitive identification of the fly must be made by an entomologist.
Control: Because these flies usually do not follow cattle into the barn, they

are difficult to control. Field control consists of spreading feces within a few days of deposit. Daily spraying with Ciodrin or dichlorvos seems to control face flies. Spray the face of each animal as it leaves the barn. Dust bags and face rubbers have also been claimed quite effective.

Selected references:

Dorsey, C. K. 1966. Face fly control experiments on quarter horses, 1962-64. *J. Econ. Entomol.* 59:86-89.

Ode, P. E., and J. G. Matthysse. 1967. Bionomics of the face fly, *Musca autumnalis* De Geer. *Memoir 402: Cornell Univ.*, Ithaca.

PARASITE: *Musca domestica* (housefly)

Disease/Infestation: Dipteriasis.

Host: An annoyance to man and animals but not a parasite in the strict sense. The larval stages may be found on fresh feces and occasionally in suppurating wounds.

Habitat: Found in association with man and animals. Female is attracted to horse manure for oviposition although pig, human, or other excrement is equally acceptable. This fly may migrate as far as 13 miles.

Identification: These are medium-size flies, to 9 mm. long. They vary from mouse-grey to dark grey and have 4 distinct longitudinal dark stripes on the thorax. The mouth parts are suited for sucking semiliquid food; there are no mandibles and maxillae. The labium is expanded into 2 labellae that can transfer fluids and semifluids.

Distribution and importance: Generally distributed wherever man and other animals are found throughout the temperate zones. Houseflies are of great medical and veterinary medical importance as mechanical vectors of many helminth, protozoan, bacterial, and viral infections.

Life cycle: This insect undergoes complete metamorphosis. Under summer conditions, the life cycle is as follows: After oviposition the creamy-white, banana-shaped egg (about 1 mm. long) hatches in 6-12 hours under optimum conditions. The egg is not resistant to drying, and few appear to survive temperatures above 40°C. or below 15°C. Larval development may occur in a few days to 3 weeks, depending on the temperature and availability of food. Optimum temperature for larval development is about 36°C. The larva then becomes a pupa in about 6 hours. The pupa persists 4-5 days in warm weather. After the adult emerges, it flies searching for food and copulates after a few days. The usual length of the life cycle is about 3 weeks, though development from egg to adult has been observed to occur in 10.4 days at 30°C. In temperate climates it is thought that the fly overwinters as a pupa.

Transmission: Flies from one animal to another.

Signs and pathogenicity: The role of the ubiquitous housefly as a vector of organisms pathogenic to man and domestic animals has been known for many years. The housefly also serves as an intermediate host for several protozoan and helminth parasites and as a mechanical vector for pathogenic bacteria and viruses. It is an important vector owing to its morphological structure, feeding habits, and close association with man and domestic animals.

Control: Control is based on general sanitation and adoption of a mangement program of collection, treatment, or disposal of manure and garbage so that fly breeding is minimal. An insecticide such as pyrethrum combined with a synergist to enhance its action destroys adults. Appropriate chlorinated hydrocarbons or organic phosphate formulations should be used for control by residual action.

Selected references:

Greenberg, B. 1965. Flies and Disease. *Scientific American* 213:92-99.
——. 1973. *Flies and Disease. Vol. 2.* Princeton: Princeton University Press.
West, L. S. 1951. *The housefly: Its natural history, medical importance, and control.* Ithaca: Comstock.

PARASITE: *Oestrus ovis* (nose bot, sheep nose-fly, grub-in-the-head, sheep gad-fly)

Disease/Infestation: Nasal myiasis.

Host: Sheep, goat, and rarely man.

Habitat: Adult flies are most active during the summer. In early morning and late afternoon they rest in the sun on the side of a water tank, a sunny barn door, a fly screen, or other object in direct sunlight. Larvae are deposited around the nostrils of the host. They crawl in and are found in the nasal passages and frontal and nasal sinuses.

Identification: The adult fly, about 12 mm. long, is grey-brown and has many small black spots on the thorax. The larva is white, yellow, and brown with dark transverse bands on the dorsal surface of the segments. The color varies with the stage of development. The larva may be 25-30 mm. long.

Distribution and importance: Generally found throughout the U.S. where sheep are raised. It may be an annoying and worrisome pest for a flock, and if brain tissue is invaded, fatalities may result.

Life cycle: The female produces larvae and may deposit as many as 60 on the sheep's nostrils in 1 hour. The larva then crawls up and enters the nasal and frontal sinuses. The rate of development of the 1st larval instar varies from 2 weeks to 9 months during during cold weather. The full-grown larva crawls out of the nose in the spring and pupates on the ground for 3-9 weeks depending on environmental conditions. After hatching, the adult fly lives approximately 2 weeks.

Transmission: Flies attack actively during the hottest part of the day.

Signs and pathogenicity: During periods of fly attack, the host stops eating and becomes restless. It shakes its head and holds its nose close to the ground. Animals often form a circle with their heads toward the center. Sneezing, head-shaking, and stomping with front feet are common indications that the flies are attacking. Activity of the larva in the nasal passages causes thickening of the nasal mucosa, mucopurulent discharge (snotty nose), and impaired respiration. Larvae that enter the sinuses may occasionally reach the brain with fatal results. Flies are annoying and cause interrupted feeding and inadequate rest. The adult fly does not bite or sting.

Diagnosis: Usually made tentatively by observing the behavior of the host in the field during the season of fly attack. Snotty nose and the demonstration of a larva expelled by sneezing are helpful in arriving at a diagnosis.

Control: Fly repellents are short-lived and have not proved satisfactory. Smearing the nose with pine-tar has frequently been recommended, but it has not been shown of any real value. Injection of 3% saponified cresol at 35-40 lb. pressure, 1 fluid ounce for each nostril, has been claimed effective. This fall and early winter treatment is directed against the 1st-stage larva in the nasal passages. Ruelene given orally as a drench should provide satisfactory control.

Selected references:

Cobbett, N. G. 1940. A method of large scale treatment of sheep for the destruction of head grubs (*Oestrus ovis*). *J. Am. Vet. Med. Assoc.* 97:571-75.

Drummond, R. O. 1966. Systemic insecticides to control larvae of *Oestrus ovis*. *J. Parasitol.* 52:192-95.

Rogers, C. E., and F. W. Knapp. 1973. Bionomics of the sheep botfly. *Envir. Ent.* 2: 11-23.

PARASITE: Species of *Phormia*, *Lucilia*, and *Calliphora* (blowflies, fleece worms, green bottles, blue bottles)

Disease/Infestation: Cutaneous myiasis, fly strike.

Host: Sheep, cattle, and other mammals.

Habitat: Flies are attracted by dead, soiled, or decomposing tissue, carrion, scraps, and putrifying waste such as domestic garbage. Larvae are found feeding on dead animals as well as other decomposing organic material.

Identification: The identification of adult flies is probably best left to the specialist. A preliminary determination may be made on the basis of the metallic coloring of the adults. In the larval stages the characteristics of spiracular plates and the cephalopharyngeal skeleton are used in identification.

Distribution and importance: Widely distributed throughout the U.S. and a serious economic problem in sheep- and cattle-raising areas.

Life cycle: The newly emerged female fly seeks a meal of animal protein, and after copulation, eggs are laid in 5-7 days. In summer the larva hatches in 6-48 hours and is full grown, about 12 mm. long, in 3-9 days. Pupation requires 3-7 days, and the adult emerges in about 11 days. The complete life cycle requires 16-35 days; the average is about 22 days. Rate of development depends on climatic conditions and the availability of food.

Transmission: Adult flies are attracted by decomposing tissue and fly from one source to another.

Signs and pathogenicity: Affected animals become depressed, stand with their heads down, do not feed, and attempt to bite infected areas. Examination of the animal shows an area of dirty moist wool or hair with a nauseating odor. The maggots attack the skin and cause its decomposition. They may form deep tunnels in the tissues. The traumatized area discharges a foul-smelling material which permeates the surrounding wool. In sheep, fleece that is wet for long periods, skin soiled with urine, and the decomposing tissue of a contaminated wound are all attractive to the egg-laying blowfly. The first larvae developing in the lesion create a favorable medium attracting more flies. Proteolytic enzymes are secreted which digest and liquidize the host's tissues. The parasites and the decomposition products are both irritating to the host. The infected animal does not feed properly and becomes sickly. If no treatment is provided, death will follow probably as a result of generalized toxemia.

Diagnosis: Made from clinical signs and identification of larvae in decomposed and putrefying tissue.

Control: Control measures are directed toward killing the larvae in the lesions, promoting healing, and preventing reinfestation. In sheep, tagging or shearing the wool in the area around the tail and hind legs is a good preventive procedure. To prevent wound infestation, materials such as EQ 335 or 5% coumaphos dust should be applied weekly. More general prophylactic measures include wetting the wool and skin with larvicidal and insecticidal preparations such as the organic phosphates ronnel, coumaphos, and diazinon. Dipping, spraying, and the use of "run through" spray pens are among the many techniques to apply insecticides. Selective breeding, surgical removal of breech folds, crutching, and care in docking should be used for blowfly prevention. Carcasses should be burned or buried to destroy flies and eliminate breeding places.

Selected references:

Hall, D. G. 1948. *The blowflies of North America.* College Park, Md.: Thomas Say Foundation.

James, M. T. 1947. The flies that cause myiasis in man. *U. S. D. A. Misc. Pub. 631.*

Zumpt, F. 1965. Myiasis in man and animals in the Old World. London: Butterworth.

PARASITE: *Pulex irritans* (human flea), *Ctenocephalides felis* (cat flea), *Ctenocephalides canis* (dog flea)

Disease/Infestation: Aphanipterosis.

Host: Man, cat, and dog. These 3 fleas are not host specific and may attack any of the hosts available.

Habitat: Although each species may be best adapted to a particular host, many fleas, if hungry, will feed on any warm-blooded mammal available. Adult fleas may be considered temporary ectoparasites because they do not remain on the host at all times. Flea larvae are not parasitic; they are found in the bedding and sleeping quarters of the host, in cracks and crevices in the floors, and under carpets. They feed on organic debris and the blood in the feces of the adult flea.

Identification: The adult flea is compressed laterally and is 2-4 mm. long. The legs are well developed, and there are no wings. In *Ctenocephalides* the spines on the head and thorax are known as combs or ctenidia. A genal comb is present on the cheek and a pronotal comb on the posterior border of the 1st thoracic segment. In *Pulex* there are no combs. The oval egg, about 0.5 mm. long, is pearly-white. The creamy-white larva, about 6 mm. long, is segmented and hairy, each segment bearing a few long hairs.

Distribution and importance: Widely scattered throughout North America; of considerable economic importance to owners of companion animals.

Life cycle: The egg is usually deposited in dust and dirt. If it is laid on the host, it soon drops off. Depending upon temperature and humidity, the egg hatches in 2-12 days. The larva develops in 9-15 days, spins a cocoon, and pupates 10-17 days under ordinary circumstances. If conditions are adverse, the pupa may not hatch for many months. The flea frequently leaves its host, and life span varies with species and depends on whether the flea has fed on blood. If the relative humidity is high, unfed fleas may survive for several months in a cool environment. The life cycle is completed in about 1 month if temperature and relative humidity are suitable.

Transmission: Through contact with infested animals, their kennels, nests, sleeping quarters, dens, and other habitats.

Signs and pathogenicity: Fleas annoy the host, thus the host bites and scratches to rid itself of the insects. The coats of infested animals become soiled. Some dogs become hypersensitive to flea bites, and an intense pruritus may result. Discrete denuded areas or "hot spots" develop. These are difficult to treat and may result in a chronic dermatitis. Secondary infections may produce chronic pruritus. Flea dermatitis in a hypersensitive animal may prove difficult to treat.

Diagnosis: Identification of the adult from the hair coat of the host or of the adult or larva from bedding debris. Examination of the hair coat for flea feces may be helpful.

Control: To control fleas the host must be treated, and its environment must be cleaned. Infested animals are treated with washes and dusts of appropriate insecticides such as pyrethrum or rotenone. These materials are effective and safe to use. Dusts or sprays of malathion or carbaryl are also effective but should not be used on cats. Flea collars impregnated with dichlorvos will provide flea control for 3 months. Animals wearing flea collars should be examined occasionally for fur loss, allergic reaction, or any evidence of collar dermatitis. Of great importance in control is cleaning the living and sleeping quarters of the host. If a flea infestation involves the owner's home, the premises should be thoroughly cleaned with a vacuum cleaner. Movable furnishings such as rugs, mats, and bedding should be taken outdoors and aired in a dry, sunny place. An insecticide with residual activity should be dusted or sprayed along baseboards, around heavy furniture, under the edges of carpets, and in floor cracks and crevices. Any hiding places of adult fleas or larvae should be treated. For indoor use, methoxychlor, chlordane, or malathion sprays may be effective. In extremely heavy infestations, it may be necessary to employ the services of a professional exterminator. For the hypersensitive animal, desensitization with a flea antigen should be considered, though the procedure is only moderately successful.

Selected references:

Hubbard, C. A. 1947. *Fleas of western North America*. Ames: Iowa State College Press.

Muller, G. H. 1970. Flea collar dermatitis in animals. *J. Am. Vet. Med. Assoc.* 157: 1616-26.

PARASITE: *Stomoxys calcitrans* (stable fly, dog fly, biting housefly)

Disease/Infestation: Dipterosis.

Host: Many domestic animals and man.

Habitat: Usually the lower parts of the body, i.e., the limbs and belly. In man they often attack the area around the ankles, and in the dog the ears are frequently bitten.

Identification: Closely resembles the housefly in general appearance and size. It is dark grey, and the head has a slender, rigid proboscis which projects and is readily seen. The grey thorax has 4 longitudinal, dark stripes.

Distribution and importance: Widely distributed throughout North America; very important because the flies breed in piles of sea and lake weeds. They may become so annoying to man that beaches or resorts may temporarily close.

Life cycle: Before oviposition, the female needs 1 or more blood meals. The eggs are deposited singly or in clumps in moist and rotting straw, piles of grass or grass clippings, and espeically on weeds washed up along the beaches. The female may deposit about 600 eggs. Each creamy-white egg is elongate, and hatches in 1-3 days. In warm weather the larva may be fully grown in 14-24 days. The adult fly emerges from the pupa in about 6-9 days depending on relative humidity and temperature. The pupa is about 6-7 mm. long. The entire life cycle is completed in about 12-30 days. The life span of the adult has been reported as about 20-69 days.

Transmission: Flies from one host to the next to feed.

Signs and pathogenicity: The adult feeds diurnally, seeking a host in both cloudy and clear weather. The bite is painful to livestock, and the puncture wound may bleed freely. Decrease in milk production, weight loss, and blood loss may all be observed when large numbers of flies attack. In the dog, the bend of the ear is frequently attacked. The area becomes traumatized and raw and may become infected. This fly serves as an intermediate host for the stomach worm of horses, *Habronema microstoma*.

Control: Because the fly generally visits the host for only short periods, the usual spray protection procedures are not highly effective. Spraying the resting places of the fly, such as fences and walls around the barnyard, is helpful. Barns should be fogged with an acceptable insecticide. Sanitation and the elimination of breeding places are extremely important.

Selected references:

Simmons, S. W. 1944. Observations on the biology of the stable fly in Florida. *J. Econ. Entomol.* 37:680-86.

Simmons, S. W., and W. E. Dove. 1941. Breeding places of the stable fly or "dog fly" *Stomoxys calcitrans* (L.) in northwestern Florida. *J. Econ. Entomol.* 34:457-62.

PARASITE: *Tabanus* spp. (horsefly, gadflies, greenheads, clegs), *Chrysops* spp. (deerfly)

Disease/Infestation: Dipterosis.

Host: Horses, cattle, deer, and sometimes man.

Habitat: Adults generally feed outdoors and do not enter the human abodes or animal shelters in search of hosts. Most species are active in the early morning or late afternoon. After ingesting a full blood meal, the female rests on the underside of a leaf or stone or on the side of a nearby building.

Identification: Robust flies, about 25 mm. long, with heavy bodies, powerful wings, and large eyes. Many are highly colored. Deerflies (*Chrysops*) are medium-size. The wings are banded, and the yellow to brown abdomen has black patches and longitudinal bands.

Distribution and importance: Widespread where water is abundant. Production losses are due principally to annoyance and blood loss. Flies consume 0.1-0.3 ml. blood at a feeding. The fly may also serve as a mechanical vector for the causal agents of anthrax, tularemia, and equine infectious anemia.

Life cycle: Eggs are laid near water on leaves, overhanging vegetation, sticks, and stones. Each torpedo-shaped egg, 1-2 mm. long, is coated with a waterproof protective substance. The egg is usually creamy-white but may darken with age. The larva is usually found in shallow water, moist soil, or wet mud at the edge of swamps, sloughs, and shallow ponds. The duration of the larval stage is variable but quite long; it may be 1 year or more. The larva transforms into a brown pupa, 10-37 mm. long. The pupal stage spans a few days to 2 weeks. The life cycle may be completed in 3-5 months but usually extends 1 year in temperate climates.

Transmission: The adult flies from host to host to obtain a blood meal.

Signs and pathogenicity: Bites are painful and irritating, and animals under attack to do not rest or feed properly. If in harness, they become unmanageable. Milk production may drop 50% at the height of the fly season.

Diagnosis: Adult flies are recognized by their size, powerful wings, and large compound eyes.

Control: It is very difficult to control this bloodsucking fly. Repellents such as synergized pyrethrum seem to provide the best results. They must be applied every 2-3 days, often more frequently in fly season.

Selected references:

Philip, C. B. 1931. The Tabanidae (horseflies) of Minnesota with special reference to their biologies and taxonomy. *Minn. Tech. Bul. 80.*

Stone, A. 1938. The horseflies of the subfamily Tabaninae of the Neoarctic Region. *U.S.D.A. Misc. Pub. 305.*

PARASITE: *Trichodectes canis* (chewing louse), *Heterodoxus* sp. (chewing louse), *Felicola subrostrata* (chewing louse of cats), *Linognathus setosus* (sucking louse)

Disease/Infestation: Phthirapterosis.

Host: Dog, cat.

Habitat: Skin.

Identification: *T. canis* is small, about 1.5 mm. long. The anterior and lateral margins of the broad head are well rounded. *Heterodoxus* sp. is about 2 mm. long; the head is roughly triangular and somewhat pointed. *F. subrostrata* varies from less than 1.0 to 1.2 mm. long. *L. setosus* is about 1.5 mm. long; it is bluish when fully fed.

Distribution and importance: All species are widely distributed throughout North America.

Life cycle: The life history of lice is essentially the same for all species although there are some minor variations in the development of individual stages (See life cycle under *Bovicola* spp. and *Haematopinus* spp.).

Transmission: Usually by contact with infested individuals but also by use of contaminated combs, brushes, blankets, and other equipment.

Signs and pathogenicity: Lousiness in dogs and cats is frequently overlooked. Infested animals scratch incessantly, day and night. Individuals heavily infested with sucking lice become weak, emaciated, and anemic. In addition to its role as a pest, *T. canis* may serve as an intermediate host for the double-pored tapeworm, *Dipylidium caninum*. In addition to good husbandry, nutrition of the host seems to be important in the control of lice. Well-nourished animals are not as likely to have heavy infestations as poorly cared for, ill-nourished individuals.

Diagnosis: Identification of individuals collected directly from the hair coat. The presence of nits is often helpful in making a diagnosis. They can be recognized by using a magnifying lens and a good light or by examining infested hairs under a low-magnification dissecting microscope.

Control: A well-balanced diet with an adequate vitamin B_2 source appears to be important in the control of lice. If the owner agrees and weather conditions are suitable, clipping can be employed to remove many lice and nits. Many excellent proprietary products are available for controlling lice on dogs and cats. Animals may be dusted with insecticides such as derris, pyrethrum, and other suitable powders. If using dusts, treatments should be repeated at 10-day to 2-week intervals until the pest is controlled. Dips are widely used for dogs; this treatment probably must be repeated after 2 weeks because most dip compounds do not kill nits.

PARASITE: *Wohlfahrtia vigil* (flesh fly)

Disease/Infestation: Cutaneous myiasis.

Host: Young dogs, foxes, mink, and children.

Habitat: Larvae are laid on and penetrate the tender skin of the newborn. The larvae usually are unable to penetrate the skin of older individuals. Adult flies feed on nectar-bearing flowers and weeds.

Identification: The adult fly is seldom seen. It is more robust than the blow-fly and has a light-grey abdomen checkered with grey and black circular spots. In some species the abdomen may appear almost entirely black.

Distribution and importance: Widespread throughout northern areas of the U.S. It is an important pest of ranched mink and foxes in the North Central and Rocky Mountain regions of the U.S.

Life cycle: The length of the life cycle is variable but usually is 30-36 days. The larva develops in 7-9 days, the pupa in 10-12 days. The adult fly deposits larvae 11-17 days after emergence.

Transmission: Female flies enter kennels and nest boxes to deposit larvae. The flies do not rest on the equipment but lay larvae directly on the newborn host.

Signs and pathogenicity: The larva is capable of penetrating the skin of the newborn. An abscess or boillike lesion several millimeters in diameter develops. Usually 1 larva is found per lesion, though 4 or 5 have been found in a boil. Parasitized animals lose condition, are feverish and markedly irritable, become dehydrated, and eat less.

Diagnosis: By the characteristic boillike lesion, age of the host, and identification of the larva.

Control: The larva generally may be removed from the lesion by gentle pressure. A small amount of chloroform or ether applied to the opening of the lesion may be helpful before removing the larva with forceps. The wound should be disinfected. A teaspoon of ronnel can be placed in the bedding of the nest box as a control measure. This may be repeated in a couple of weeks. Ronnel should not be used in the bedding of kits less than 3 days old.

Selected references:

Eschle, J. L., and G. R. DeFoliart. 1965a. Control of mink myiasis caused by the larvae of *Wohlfahrtia vigil*. *J. Econ. Entomol.* 58:529-31.

———. 1965b. Rearing and biology of *Wohlfahrtia vigil* (Diptera; Sarcophagidae). *Ann. Entom. Soc. Amer.* 58:849-55.

C. Linguatulids

PARASITE: *Linguatula serrata* (tongue worm, pentastome)

Disease/Infestation: Linguatulosis.

Host: Dog, fox, wolf.

Habitat: Nasal and respiratory passages.

Identification: This peculiar group of wormlike arthropods is related to the mites. The adults are internal parasites of nasal and respiratory organs of vertebrates. They are frequently tongue shaped and have an annulated cuticle which makes the body appear segmented. The female is 8-13 cm. long and the male, 1.2-2.0 cm. long. The yellow egg, about 90 x 70 μ, is oval and contains a larva bearing 4 hooklike structures. The head is not distinctly separated from the body. The anterior end has 5 ventral protuberances. The median opens into the mouth, and chitinous hooks protrude from the remaining 4.

Distribution and importance: Widely distributed but not commonly recorded from domestic animals.

Life cycle: The eggs are expelled from the respiratory tract and are swallowed by one of a wide variety of herbivorous intermediate hosts such as the sheep, rabbit, cow, horse, and other mammals, including man. The larva hatches in the intestine of the intermediate host, penetrates the intestinal wall, finds its way to the lymphatic or blood vessels, and is then transported to various visceral organs such as the lymph glands, liver, lungs, and kidney. The minute, 4-hooked larva is encapsulated by the host but continues to develop. After several molts over 4-6 months, it becomes an infective nymph, 4-6 mm. long. The infective nymph may remain alive in the intermediate host for several months or even years.

Transmission: Many methods of transmission have been suggested. At present about all that can be said is that the carnivore acquires the parasite by ingestion of the intermediate host infected with the young parasite.

Signs and pathogenicity: In the definitive host, signs are variable depending on the number of worms present and their location. The parasites attach to the nasal mucosa and may cause some irritation and mechanical blockage of the nasal passages. Animals are said to sneeze and cough intermittently and may rub their noses with the forefeet. A blood-stained nasal discharge is occasionally seen.

Diagnosis: By noting the clinical signs, finding the characteristic eggs in the nasal discharge and feces, or by directly observing the parasite in the posterior nasal passages.

Control: Infections may be avoided if carnivores are prevented from eating infected viscera of one of the many intermediate hosts. The use of parasiticides has not proved effective. Surgical trephining and removal of the parasite has proven feasible.

Selected references:

Penn, G. H. 1942. The life history of *Porocephalus crotali*, a parasite of the Louisiana muskrat. *J. Parasitol.* 28:277-83.

Sambon, L. W. 1922. A synopsis of the family Linguatulidae. *J. Trop. Med. and Hyg.* 25:188-206, 391-428.

APPENDIXES

Appendix A
Parasitological Laboratory
Techniques and Diagnostic Procedures

There is no single best method for collection and preservation of parasites. Each individual prefers certain techniques and procedures, and simple general procedures may be modified for specific use in both the field and laboratory. The availability and condition of material for examination, the size of the parasites, and the physical facilities at one's disposal are all important considerations in choosing an appropriate procedure. Final diagnosis of a parasitic infection or infestation depends on specific identification of the parasite, which in many instances can be made only in the laboratory. To aid the taxonomist, specimens should be collected and preserved in the best possible condition so that morphologic structures and details can be seen to best advantage.

ECTOPARASITES

When the carcass is examined for external lesions, a thorough search should be made for adults, eggs, and larvae of ectoparasites. Although most ectoparasites leave the body at death, a few specimens may remain as evidence of antemortem infestation. The external parasites of most domestic animals are ticks, fleas, lice, and mites. With the exception of mites, these arthropods can be seen readily by the careful observer.

Examination of individual large domestic animals is usually limited to gross examination of the hair or wool for adults or their eggs, usually with the unaided eye or a flashlight with built-in magnifying lens. If specimens are seen, they should be picked off, dropped into a vial containing 70% ethyl alcohol, and appropriately labeled with host, geographic location, habitat on host, date, and name of the collector.

Ticks

Engorged ticks may be anchored firmly to the skin of the live animal and may remain there some time after death of the host. To remove the tick, grasp it gently with a pair of forceps and maintain continuous tension until the tick releases its hold. A drop or two of chloroform or ether on the live tick may hasten detachment. Probably the most commonly used fixative and preservative is 70% alcohol; it is usually available.

Fleas and Lice

These insects may be collected by using forceps or touching the parasites with a small camel's-hair brush that has been moistened with alcohol or xylene. A small animal can be examined by placing it on a sheet of paper and combing the hair. Collect insects from the paper and preserve in 70% alcohol.

Mites

In examining the ear for mites, sufficient exudate can usually be collected to find many mites. Scabs and exudative crusts may be dropped in 70% alcohol and examined later for mites. In mange in which burrowing mites are suspected, deep skin scrapings should be made.

Skin Scraping

- Place a drop of mineral oil on a clean, glass slide.
- Dip a clean, blunt scalpel in the oil drop and make a deep skin scraping (until petechial hemorrhage appears if you seek burrowing mites) at the edge of the lesion.
- Transfer scraped material to the oil on the slide and mix gently.
- Place a cover glass on the oil and debris and press lightly.
- With the light much reduced, examine the scraping at 100 x magnification of the microscope. The mites will be transparent and, if motile, easily seen wallowing in the oily medium.

Some larger mites, especially those that do not burrow, may be seen readily by placing the debris from a skin scraping on black paper. Under a light the mites appear as actively moving white specks.

If the initial scraping proves negative, more scrapings should be taken. One may have to use a digestion-maceration procedure, including sedimentation or centrifugal concentration of mites.

Alkali Digestion and Maceration Procedure

- Make a liberal skin scraping without using oil.
- Place material in a test tube or small beaker.
- Cover with a 5-10% solution of sodium or potassium hydroxide.
- Allow to macerate overnight or heat gently for 5 minutes.

—Add water and allow mixture to stand until sediment is seen in bottom of container. (To hasten sedimentation, centrifugation may be used.)

—Take a sample of sediment with medicine dropper or pipette, transfer to a slide, place a coverslip on the slide, and examine at 100 x magnification.

Ectoparasites of Birds and Small Mammals

Collection of fleas, lice, and mites from small mammals and birds is best accomplished by brushing, combing, or shaking the fur, hair, or feathers over a white tray or large sheet of white paper. The ectoparasites can then be collected with forceps or a fine camel's-hair brush moistened with alcohol. They should be permanently stored in 70% alcohol. If examining a small mammal or bird expressly to collect ectoparasites, the freshly killed specimen should be placed in a light paper, finely woven cotton, or polyethylene bag, and the bag should be securely tied. As the host cools, the ectoparasites leave the animal and can be seen on examination of the debris in the bag.

An alternative method is to immerse the host in a small pail of water containing a detergent. The skin surface is cleaned, and any ectoparasites present are liberated. After agitating the specimen, remove it and allow the wash water to sediment or pour the wash water through a fine wire strainer or bolting cloth. Examine the collected material for ectoparasites. Larval arthropods, such as fly larvae, are best preserved in 70% alcohol; 5% formalin is a second choice.

ENDOPARASITES

Parasites within the host should should be collected systematically. Although parasites may be found in almost any organ or tissue of the host, blood, muscle, the trachea, lung, stomach, intestines, liver, heart, and kidneys are most frequently infected. Parasites are found not only in the lumen of an organ but also deeply embedded in the tissue parenchyma. Careful examination and dissection are necessary, and tissue sections often reveal interesting parasites.

If possible, blood smears should be examined for protozoa and microfilariae. Of the many methods available for staining blood, Wright's and Giemsa stains are probably the most satisfactory for routine use.

Intestinal Protozoa

Material to be examined for protozoa should be as fresh as possible and should be left in the intestinal fluid. Trophozoites are seldom found in the digestive tracts of animals that have been dead any length of time. The material in direct smears, if taken from the digestive tract, may be mixed with a little warm saline and examined immediately for motile trophozoites.

Many protozoans of the gastrointestinal tract live in fluid or soft feces, and to observe these stages the feces must be examined immediately. If a specimen cannot be examined immediately, place it in a prewarmed glass container that can, in turn, be placed in another container holding water at body temperature. Widemouthed thermos bottles may also be used for this purpose. Protozoan cysts are far less delicate and may be recognized several days after passage, especially if the sample has been refrigerated (See Examination of Feces).

Helminths

Collection of Helminths

Choice of method depends on the necropsy and laboratory facilities available. In the field the knife is probably the only available instrument, whereas a more thorough and detailed parasitological examination is possible in the laboratory.

1. Field Collection of Helminths. The equipment is simple and generally available. Sharp knives, cord, labels, pails, a pyrex pie plate, specimen jars, and preserving fluids are all essential.

On routine necropsy, the digestive tract parasites are most frequently encountered. The viscera should be opened and the mucosal surfaces examined for lesions and helminths. If a detailed examination for parasites is indicated, tissue and organs may be refrigerated, frozen, or preserved in formalin and examined later in the laboratory.

Small animals or birds may be preserved in toto in a garbage can containing 10% formalin solution. To allow adequate fixation, a slit should be made through the abdominal wall to expose the viscera to the fixative.

If examination of larger animals must be delayed, only the viscera need be saved. If feasible, before preserving the viscera a piece of string should be tied at the junction of the esophagus and stomach, the pyloric sphincter, the ileocecal valve, the cecocolonic junction, and the rectum. This practice helps retain the parasites in their normal habitats and facilitates identification.

General information including the name of the host, location of the parasite in the host, geographic locality, and other relevant data should be written in pencil on a tag, and the tag should be tied to the set of viscera. A good quality label will remain intact, and the writing will remain legible for several months in a formalin solution. If the preserved viscera are shipped to a laboratory for examination, drain the surplus fixative, fill the shipping container with burlap or other packing material, and securely attach the lid.

An alternative to chemical preservation is freezing whole animals or viscera. If the volume of material is small, the frozen specimen should be packed inside another container and the space between the two containers filled with sawdust or some other insulating material. If dry ice is available, the material should arrive at its destination in excellent condition.

2. Laboratory Procedures for Collection of Helminths. Generally the equipment required for the collection of helminths is simple and inexpensive. Helminths may be found in almost any organ or tissue of the host. The larger worms are usually seen easily; the smaller ones may be seen with a good 4-in. diameter reading glass or a dissecting microscope. Liver and lung tissue should be sliced and smears taken directly from the cut surface and examined for eggs or larvae. The slices may then be squeezed in a dish of warm water to liberate any adult worms. Because the digestive tract harbors many different helminths, each area should be examined separately. The contents should be washed with tepid water into a small pail or glass culture dish. Examination of the contents of each organ or section of the digestive tract should be made separately because a parasite species may be limited to a particular location or habitat. The small intestine may be opened by drawing it over the blade of a sharp pair of bandage scissors. The contents of the tract may then be washed off the mucosal surface and examined.

To examine the intestine without opening it, one end is placed in a bucket, and starting at the other end, the intestine is stripped between the fingers and the lumen contents collected in a pail. As an alternative, the intestine may be slipped over a water faucet nozzle, and the lumen contents may be gently washed into a pail.

It is advantageous to remove as much coarse, undigested material as possible. This may be accomplished by either of two common procedures: simple sedimentation or washing through a graded series of metal sieves.

a. Sedimentation. Protozoan cysts, helminths, and helminth eggs sink in water and may be cleaned and concentrated by sedimentation. Some solid material from the intestines may dissolve, remain in suspension, or float to the surface. Fill the pail or can containing the contents of a single organ with water. Gently agitate the surface with a wooden applicator or glass rod and allow the suspension to settle *at least* 10 minutes. Agitation of the surface is necessary to sediment worms that may be floating on mucus, feed material, or other debris. Carefully siphon or decant the supernatant and refill the container. Repeat until a large amount of the floating debris has been removed. Finally pour the sediment into flat culture dishes (deep pyrex pie plates are suitable for this purpose) and examine over black paper, a black enamel tray, or black table top. Using forceps, pick out the helminths. It may be necessary to use a reading glass or dissecting microscope to find the smaller forms.

If it is not convenient to examine the material immediately, the sediment may be placed in an ordinary fruit jar, mixed with equal amounts of 10 percent formalin, labeled, and examined later.

b. Sieving. An alternative method that is quicker is screening and washing the material through a series of nested sieves. A very satisfactory set is the U.S. Standard Sieve Series, available in many different mesh sizes. These sieves nest tightly but can be easily separated and cleaned. Sieves are stacked with the coarsest mesh on the top. The material to be sieved is poured into the top and then washed gently through the other sieves. After thorough washing, the sieves are separated, and each is inverted over a glass culture dish or a deep pie plate and the debris washed into the dish. After sedimentation the supernatant of each dish is gently poured off and the sediment examined.

c. Retrieving Worms from Sediments. There is no shortcut in recovering worms from sediment or sieved material. Large worms can be picked up easily with forceps, but minute forms must be picked out with fine needles or forceps. The very small and delicate forms must be retrieved under about 20 x magnification of the dissecting microscope. Under the microscope, minute adults or larvae may be sucked into a pipette, transferred to a small glass dish such as a Syracuse watch glass, and preserved.

d. Collecting Nematode Larvae from Feces. Feces should be collected from the rectum of the animal to avoid contamination with free-living nematodes from the soil. For a fecal culture, feces may be mixed with an equal amount of powdered animal charcoal. Add a small amount of water to form a fairly thick paste. Spread the mixture in a thin layer over the bottom of a petri dish. Cut a piece of filter paper to fit inside the lid of the dish, insert it in the lid, and moisten it. The larvae will develop rapidly in this moist culture chamber. In a week to 10 days at room temperature and in subdued light, infective larvae migrate up the sides of the dish and congregate on the moist paper in the lid of the petri plate. The paper can be removed and the larvae washed off with water and concentrated by sedimentation or centrifugation. Because herbivorous animals produce copious feces, parasites of these hosts may best be cultured by placing the material in a glass jar (Mason), adding a little water, and covering with a loose lid. The culture should be moist enough that droplets of condensate form on the walls of the jar. If kept at room temperature in subdued light for about a week, the larvae will migrate up the walls of the jar. The larvae may be seen with a hand magnifier.

Baermann Procedure. If the larval forms of concern do not migrate from feces readily, an isolation and concentration procedure may be used. The usual method is the Baermann technique for concentration of larvae from soil or feces and for isolation of larvae from chopped lung, liver, or other tissues suspected of harboring nematode larvae. The Baermann procedure is based on the principle that most larvae migrate from feces or tissue into warm water, and because they are heavier than water, they sink to the bottom of the container. The apparatus required for this technique is simple and consists of a glass funnel about 20 cm. in diameter, a rack or stand, a piece of rubber tubing, a pinch-cock, a piece of wire screen, and cheesecloth. The rubber tubing is slipped onto the stem of the funnel and clamped shut with the pinch-cock. The funnel is placed in a ringstand, and a piece of wire screen is cut to fit the widest part of the funnel. (A large sieve or gravy strainer may be used in place of the screen.) If most of the solid material is to be retained, place a layer of cheesecloth on the wire screen or sieve. Place the cultured feces on the cheesecloth, which in turn rests on the wire gauze. Pour warm water, at about 40°C., down the side of the funnel (not directly through the funnel) until the water is in contact with the cultured feces.

The warm water activates the larvae, and they sink and are concentrated in the stem of the funnel. Most larvae sediment about 1 hour after standing. Open the pinch-cock carefully and withdraw a few milliliters of fluid. Most larvae will be in the first few milliliters that are withdrawn. They may be examined immediately in a dish or concentrated by centrifugation and then examined.

3. Collection of Intermediate Hosts. One may wish to collect potential intermediate hosts, such as arthropods, mollusks, birds, and mammals. To collect a bloodsucking insect invert a widemouthed jar over it when it is feeding or resting. Fleas, ticks, lice, and mites are best collected by the techniques mentioned earlier.

It is usually desirable to collect suspected intermediate hosts alive. Preservatives may be necessary if the specimens must be mailed or if they cannot be mailed alive.

Gastropods are frequently needed for laboratory studies in connection with trematode life cycles. The help of a taxonomist is usually required for specific identification. If shipped alive, mollusks should be packed in moist moss and kept cool. For permanent preservation, the most suitable solution is 70% ethyl alcohol.

Laboratory Procedures for the Preservation of Helminths

In general, complicated fixatives are not necessary to preserve helminths unless detailed histologic and cytologic studies are anticipated. Formalin and alcohol are the most widely used preservatives.

1. Nematodes (Roundworms). Lungworms and filarial worms excepted, most nematodes may be killed and fixed satisfactorily in hot 70% ethyl alcohol. Before fixation, worms should be washed in warm physiological saline.

If dead when collected, the nematodes may be fixed in 5% formalin and later transferred to 70% ethyl alcohol. Large worms like *Ascaris* may be fixed and stored in 5 or 10% formalin. The usual storage fluid for nematodes is 70% alcohol to which is added 5% glycerin. The glycerin is a safeguard against evaporation of the alcohol; a dried helminth is of little value. Filaria and lungworms, dead or alive, tend to rupture on fixation. A satisfactory fixative for these forms is 5% formol saline; they should be stored permanently in alcohol.

After fixation, smaller species of nematodes may be cleared for microscopic examination by placing them overnight in lactophenol solution. They may be transferred to this clearing medium directly from water, formalin, or alcohol and after examination may be returned to the original preservative. Lactophenol solution consists of 1 part each of phenol, lactic acid, and water and 2 parts of glycerin.

2. Trematodes (Flukes). Probably the best general fixative for flatworms (flukes and tapeworms) is 5% formal-saline; for special studies other fixatives are available. Large flukes may be fixed under gentle pressure between glass slides. Use rubber bands to maintain pressure. Pieces of glass or toothpicks may be inserted between the slides and adjusted until the pressure is suitable. The flukes between the slides are then placed in a dish of fixative. After a few hours, the top slide is removed to allow better penetration of the fixing fluid. Small flukes may be dropped directly into 5% formol saline and stored in 70% alcohol to which 5% glycerin has been added.

Identification of flukes and tapeworms usually depends on study of their morphological characteristics. Staining of the internal structures of these helminths is necessary. For best staining results, a more complex fixative such as Gilson's, Bouin's, or Zenker's solution is suggested.

3. Cestodes (Tapeworms). It is important that cestodes be collected with the scolices attached because the latter are necessary for any taxonomic study. Freshly collected, complete worms should be placed in a dish of warm saline and allowed to relax for an hour or so. To prevent shrinkage on fixing, they may be wound around glass tubes or plates and then placed in a fixative. Five % formol-saline is a satisfactory fixative, though special fixatives may be required to show the details of morphology. They may be stored in formalin-glycerin or alcohol glycerin solution.

4. Tissue Containing Helminths. Organs and tissues containing helminths for tissue section study should be fixed in 10% formalin solution. Special fixatives used are Bouin's, Zenker's and others of the individual's choice. Corrosive sublimate, a component of some fixatives, must be removed with iodine and carefully washed before tissues can be stained or permanently preserved.

5. Preparation of Museum Specimens. The preparation of gross, museum specimens showing the helminths in situ is difficult and time-consuming. To retain natural color, Kaiserling's, Klotz's, or Jore's method of preparation of museum specimens may be tried. These methods require laboratory facilities; the results obtained are quite variable.

6. Staining of Helminths. Generally nematodes are not stained for microscopic examination. Staining is possible but not very satisfactory. Nematodes may be cleared well in lactophenol or glycerin, though clearing large specimens with glycerin is a rather long process. After clearing, small specimens may be mounted satisfactorily in glycerin jelly. A cover slip is applied and sealed with a suitable sealing cement, enamel, or lacquer. Such preparations do not last indefinitely but remain in good condition for many years.

After fixation, cestodes and trematodes may be stained, dehydrated, cleared, and mounted using procedures given in most parasitology textbooks. If specimens are small enough, they may be mounted in toto. In the case of large cestodes, take a few proglottids from several different areas of the strobila. These may be pressed, stained, and mounted. Stains generally used for flukes and tapeworms are acid and alcoholic carmines and haematoxylin. The carmine stains are easier to use, and they yield consistent results. The media for permanent mounts are Canada balsam, clarite, piccolyte, and other synthetic resins.

Helminth eggs may be fixed in 10% formalin, concentrated by sedimentation or centrifugation, and mounted in glycerin or glycerin jelly. Permanent mounts of helminth eggs are generally not satisfactory.

Plastic permanent mounts of helminths and arthropods have proved quite satisfactory especially for large specimens. Such a mount is attractive, durable, and satisfactory except that the surface is easily scratched.

Examination of Feces

The laboratory procedures to demonstrate stages of parasites of diagnostic value are many and varied. All procedures have advantages and disadvantages, and few are suitable for all purposes. The choice of procedure depends on the results required and the facilities available. Only the basic routine procedures will be presented.

Collection of Specimen

The importance of properly collected, adequately labeled, fresh specimens cannot be overemphasized. A small composite sample of the stool should be placed in an ointment tin, clean glass jar, waxed paper cup with lid, or other suitable container. Plastic bags and newsprint, tissue paper, and cardboard boxes are *not* appropriate containers. If the material is examined immediately, no preservation is necessary. If the sample must be kept until the next day or sent to a laboratory, either refrigerate or add 10% formalin solution to the feces.

Gross Examination of Feces

Observe the condition of the animal's digestive tract and its diet. Not infrequently the client's history of the diet does not describe the actual constituents seen on examination of the stool of the patient. One should note the consistency, color, presence or absence of blood, state of digestion, presence of mucus or other unusual constituents, and occurrence of large helminths.

Microscopic Examination of Feces

Equipment required includes waxed paper cups (3-oz. capacity), small sieve or strainer, straight-sided vial or centrifuge tube, glass rod or small wire loop, tongue depressors, applicator sticks, glass slides, plastic cover glasses (18 mm. square), flotation fluid of choice, microscope, and light. A centrifuge is not essential.

1. Direct Smear (Temporary Wet Mount). Fresh, saline preparations are particularly useful for detecting motile trophozoites of protozoans and helminth larvae. The smear is made by taking a small particle of feces with a toothpick or, more conveniently, using feces adhering to a thermometer and transferring this to a drop of saline on a 3- x 1-inch glass slide. The sample should be mixed so that newsprint can be read through the preparation. Cover with an 18- or 22-mm. square, cover glass and examine under 100 x magnification with reduced light. Examine the slide systematically and carefully for motile protozoans (if sample is fresh), protozoan cysts, parasite eggs, and helminth larvae.

If structures resembling protozoan cysts are seen, it may be necessary to use an iodine preparation to distinguish greater morphologic detail. Prepare the iodine smear just as the saline mount, substituting iodine solution for the saline. Alternatively, allow iodine solution to run under the coverslip of the saline mount. Several iodine solutions may be used to stain protozoan cysts.

Gram's iodine and Lugol's solution are suitable. A preferable solution is modified D'Antoni's iodine, which consists of 1 gm. potassium iodide and 1.5 gm. iodine crystals dissolved in 100 ml. distilled water. The stock solution will remain in good condition several weeks. Glycogen in the cyst appears reddish-brown, the cytoplasm, yellow, and the nuclear chromatin, brown or black.

2. Concentration Methods.

a. Sedimentation. Because protozoan cysts and helminth eggs are slightly heavier than water, simple sedimentation may be used to concentrate these forms. Mix a few grams of feces with water to make a thick fecal suspension. Pour through a fine sieve, and thin the filtrate with about 50 ml. water. Allow to settle 30 minutes to 1 hour. Pour off the supernatant and resuspend in water. Debris will be floated off or dissolved each time this is done. The sediment is examined directly for protozoan cysts and worm eggs.

Use of a centrifuge will speed this procedure. Pour the fecal suspension into a 15-ml. centrifuge tube and centrifuge 1-3 minutes at about 1500-2000 r.p.m. Pour off the supernatant and examine a smear of the sediment for parasitic stages.

b. Flotation Methods. The fecal material is mixed with a solution of greater density than that of the parasite eggs or cysts. The eggs and cysts, which are heavier than water but of lower specific gravity than the flotation fluid, rise to the surface of the medium.

Simple flotation: Take about 10 gm. of feces (a portion about the size of a walnut) and mix to a soupy consistency in a paper cup. With a tongue depressor, stir through a fine sieve. Mix filtrate with about 20 cc. of any *one* of the following flotation solutions:

- Saturated sodium nitrate solution (sp. gr. 1.200)
- Zinc sulfate solution (For sp. gr. 1.180 add 37.5 gm. $ZnSO_4 \cdot 7H_2O$ or 21 gm. anhydrous $ZnSO_4$ to 100 cc. water)
- Sugar solution (1 lb. sugar and 1% or 4 cc. phenol in 12 oz. water)
- Saturated sodium chloride solution

Mix well and fill a straight-sided vial (shell vial) so that the top of the meniscus is just level with the top of the vial. Place cover glass or 3- x 1-in. slide on top of the tube and allow to stand for 30 minutes. Lift off cover glass, transfer carefully to a slide, and examine systematically for helminth eggs and protozoan cysts. If a slide has been used, turn right side up, drop on a cover glass and examine. A disposable unit for this simple flotation procedure is now available from a commercial source.

Centrifugal flotation: A centrifuge may be used to speed flotation. Mix about 10 gm. of feces to a thin paste with a small quantity of water and passed through a fine strainer. Pour the filtrate into a 15-ml. centrifuge tube and centrifuge at 1500 r.p.m. for 2-3 minutes. Pour off the supernatant and replace with zinc sulfate solution, sugar solution, or another flotation fluid. Use a wooden applicator to thoroughly mix the semisolid material in the base of the centrifuge tube with the flotation fluid. Centrifuge the suspension again for 3-4 minutes at 1500 r.p.m. After centrifugation, transfer the eggs or cysts from the surface of the fluid in the centrifuge tube to a 3- x 1-in. glass slide using a wire loop or glass rod. Place a coverslip on the slide and examine with 100 x magnification and reduced light.

For the detection of fluke eggs simple sedimentation or Riva's procedure should be used. Fluke eggs may rupture if placed in fluid of greater specific gravity than that of the eggs.

3. Egg Counts. The presence of helminth eggs in feces confirms one's suspicions that an animal harbors worms. To estimate the concentration of worm eggs in feces, quantitative, egg-counting techniques have been developed. However, even with such techniques, it has not proved possible to estimate accurately the size of the worm population from a fecal egg count. Egg counts are primarily useful in estimating worm burdens in a group of animals subject to control or eradication programs or animals used to evaluate anthelmintic efficacy.

The accuracy of the egg counts may be influenced by such factors as diurnal fluctuation in egg output, the uneven distribution of eggs throughout the feces resulting in sampling error, the amount of feces expelled, and its moisture content. A diet with a high proportion of roughage is claimed to increase egg output.

Factors influencing the significance of egg counts may be related to host resistance, which may depress egg output or may extend the prepatent period. It should be remembered that immature worms do not lay eggs yet may be highly pathogenic. Eggs of many nematode species are not readily distinguished, and a count usually includes eggs of many species, which may differ widely in fecundity and pathogenicity. Because quantitative egg counts are not widely used in clinical diagnosis of parasitism, only one of the several methods of counting eggs will be outlined.

The Stoll egg count, a reliable dilution technique, is used to determine the number of eggs per gram of feces. Weigh 4 grams of feces in a Stoll flask. Add decinormal (0.1N) sodium hydroxide to the top ring of the flask (the 60-cc. mark). Add several glass beads, close the flask with a rubber stopper, and shake the mixture vigorously for 1 minute. To remove bubbles add 1 drop amyl alcohol. With a Stoll pipette, withdraw 0.15 ml. from the center of the flask and transfer this amount to a 2- x 3-in. slide. Cover with a 22- x 40-mm.,

No. 2 cover glass. Using a mechanical stage and 100 x magnification, count all the eggs under the coverslip. The number of eggs per gram of feces is computed by multiplying the total count by 100. Two counts are made from different 4-gm. samples, and the results are averaged.

Examination of Blood for Microfilariae

In North America the filarial worm of domestic animals of major importance is *Dirofilaria immitis*, the heartworm of the dog. Diagnosis of filarial infections is based on the clinical signs observed in the host and the demonstration and identification of characteristic microfilariae in the bloodstream. This diagnosis is complicated by the presence of another filarid species in the dog, *Dipetalonema reconditum*. The adult of this nonpathogenic species lives in the connective tissues of the dog, and the microfilariae must be differentiated from those of *Dirofilaria immitis*.

Microfilariae are differentiated on the basis of the numbers present, motility, and morphology. In *Dirofilaria* infections a few to many microfilariae are present, but in *Dipetalonema* infections usually only a very few microfilariae are seen. If large numbers of microfilariae are present, a preliminary diagnosis of *D. immitis* may be made. Recall that both species may occur in the same host. The absence of microfilariae in the circulating blood does not mean that the host does not carry an infection of *D. immitis*. Microfilariae may not be demonstrated in 5-10% of infected dogs. In such cases the diagnosis must be based on the case history and the clinical signs such as coughing, tiring easily on exercise, and impeded blood circulation. Radiography may also be of considerable value. (See *Dipetalonema* and *Dirofilaria* sections for comparison of motility, morphology, and size of the microfilariae.)

Several excellent laboratory techniques are now available for demonstrating microfilariae. Concentration procedures that kill and fix the microfilariae permit accurate measurement and morphologic study. In routine practice, the technique most widely used for detection and identification of microfilariae is the modified Knott's technique. This method is simple, quickly and easily performed, and gives fairly uniform results.

Modified Knott's Technique

Withdraw 1 ml. blood and add to 10 ml. 2% formalin in water. Immediately invert tube several times to insure thorough mixing and lysing of the blood. Centrifuge 5 minutes at 1000-1500 r.p.m. Pour off and discard the supernatant. Add 2-3 drops 1:1000 aqueous methylene blue solution to the centrifuge tube. Use a clean wooden applicator to gently mix fluid with the button of solid debris at the bottom of the tube. Allow material to stain about 5 minutes. Examine the sediment from the centrifuge tube for dead, fixed, and lightly stained microfilariae.

Direct Smear

To observe motility, place several drops of freshly drawn blood on a glass slide and place a cover glass on it. Examine *immediately* under 100 x magnification to observe the motility and numbers of microfilariae present.

Saponin Concentration Technique

Prepare a solution of 2% saponin and 2% sodium citrate in distilled water. Withdraw 1 ml. blood and add to 5-10 ml. of the saponin citrate solution. Mix well to insure complete hemolysis. Place mixture in a 15-ml. centrifuge tube and centrifuge for 1-3 minutes at 1500 r.p.m. Under 100 x magnification, examine the sediment from the tip of the centrifuge tube for the presence of living microfilariae.

For detailed information concerning filter techniques and vital staining, see the publications of Wylie (1973), Sawyer, Rubin, and Jackson (1965), and Chalifoux and Hunt (1971).

CALIBRATION OF THE MICROSCOPE

Because size is an important criterion in identification of parasites, it is important to know how to measure microscopic objects. It is frequently necessary to measure eggs, cysts, and the lengths and widths of various minute morphological structures.

The microscope must be calibrated. Two scales are necessary, an ocular or eyepiece micrometer and a stage micrometer. The former is a glass disc that is etched with a scale of 50 arbitrary divisions. The stage micrometer (a 3- x 1-in. glass slide) is etched with an absolute scale of 2 mm., usually with 0.1- and 0.01-mm. subdivisions. The exact value of the units of each ocular micrometer varies with different eyepiece and objective combinations and with different microscopes. The value of 1 unit on the ocular micrometer must be calculated for every combination of eyepiece and objective lenses. To calibrate the eyepiece micrometer, units are compared with a scale of known dimensions, those of the stage micrometer. This is accomplished by superimposing the image of the arbitrary ocular scale on the calibrated scale on the stage micrometer.

The procedure of calibration is as follows: Remove the 10x ocular from the microscope and unscrew the top lens. Place the micrometer disc on the shelf within the ocular with the etched side down. Replace the top lens and insert the ocular in the microscope. Place the stage micrometer on the stage and bring both scales into focus. Adjust the two scales so that the zero line on the ocular scale is exactly superimposed upon the zero line on the stage micrometer. Look to the right and find another place where two other lines are exactly superimposed. Because each large division of the stage micrometer is 0.1 mm. (100 μ) long, the total distance in millimeters between the two points of superimposition can be determined. Note the number of small ocular micrometer units needed to cover the same distance. For example, if 40 small divisions on the ocular micrometer equal 8 (0.8 mm.) large units on the stage, then 1 ocular unit is 0.02 mm. (or 20 μ) long.

Measurements may be expressed in millimeters or microns. Because 1 millimeter equals 1000 microns, the millimeter determination multiplied by 1000 yields the measurement in microns:

$$0.02 \text{ mm. x } 1000 = 20 \text{ microns } (\mu)$$

For reference, the values for 1 to 50 units of the ocular micrometer can be recorded in chart form. Then the size of any object can be quickly calculated by measuring it with the calibrated eyepiece micrometer.

Selected references:

Chalifoux, L., and D. D. Hunt. 1971. Histochemical differentiation of *Dirofilaria immitis* and *Dipetalonema reconditum*. *J. Amer. Vet. Med. Assoc.* 158:601-5.

Kelly, J. D. 1973. Detection and differentiation of microfilariae in canine blood. *Austral. Vet. Jour.* 49:23-27.

Ministry of Agriculture, Fisheries, and Food. 1977. Manual of veterinary parsitological laboratory technics. Tech. Bul. 18. London: Her Majesty's Stationery Office.

Sawyer, T. K., E. F. Rubin, and R. F. Jackson. 1965. The cephalic hook in microfilariae of *Dipetalonema reconditum* in the differentiation of canine filariasis. *Proc. Helm. Soc. Wash.* 32:15-20.

Sloss, M. W. 1970. *Veterinary Clinical Parasitology.* Ames: Iowa State Univ. Press.

Stein, F. J., and G. W. Lawton. 1973. Comparison of methods for diagnosis and differentiation of canine filariasis. *J. Amer. Vet. Med. Assoc.* 163:140-41.

Wylie, J. P. 1973. Detection of microfilariae by a filter technique. *J. Amer. Vet. Med. Assoc.* 156:1403-05.

Appendix B
Parasites Arranged by Host

This table includes only the parasites mentioned in the handbook; it is not a complete listing of parasites of domestic animals of North America.

Group	Location	Species
	Horse, Mule, and Donkey	
Protozoans	Digestive system	*Entamoeba coli*
		E. gedoelsti
		Tritrichomonas equi
	Circulatory system	*Babesia caballi*
		B. equi
	Skin and subcutaneous tissues	*Besnoitia besnoiti*
		Trypanosoma equiperdum
	Urogenital system	*Trypanosoma equiperdum*
	Muscle and tendon	*Sarcocystis* sp.
Nematodes	Digestive system	*Craterostomum* sp.
		Gyalocephalus sp.
		Habronema (Draschia) megastoma
		H. microstoma
		H. muscae
		Oesophagodontus sp.
		Oxyuris equi
		Parascaris equorum
		Probstmayria vivipara
		Strongyloides westeri
		Strongylus edentatus
		S. equinus
		S. vulgaris
		Trichonema spp.
		Trichostrongylus axei
		Triodontophorus spp.
	Respiratory system	*Dictyocaulus arnfieldi*
		Micronema deletrix
	Skin and subcutaneous tissues	*Onchocerca cervicalis*
		Habronema spp.
	Serous cavities	*Setaria equina*

Parasites Arranged by Host (Continued)

Group	Location	Species
Cestodes	Digestive system	*Anoplocephala magna*
		A. perfoliata
		Paranoplocephala mamillana
Arachnids	Skin and subcutaneous tissues	*Chorioptes equi*
		Dermacentor albipictus
		D. variabilis
		Otobius megnini
		Psoroptes equi
		Sarcoptes scabiei var. *equi*
Insects	Digestive system	*Gasterophilus hemorrhoidalis*
		G. intestinalis
		G. nasalis
	Skin and subcutaneous tissues	*Bovicola equi*
		Chrysops sp.
		Cochliomyia (Callitroga) hominivorax
		Haematopinus asini
		Hypoderma spp.
		Stomoxys calcitrans
		Tabanus spp.

Cattle

Group	Location	Species
Protozoans	Digestive system	*Eimeria auburnensis*
		E. bovis
		E. zurnii
		Entamoeba bovis
	Circulatory system	*Babesia bigemina*
		Theileria sp.
		Trypanosoma theileri (americanum)
	Muscle and tendon	*Sarcocystis* sp.
	Skin and subcutaneous tissues	*Besnoitia besnoiti*
	Reproductive system	*Tritrichomonas foetus*
	Miscellaneous tissues	*Toxoplasma gondii*
Nematodes	Digestive system	*Bunostomum phlebotomum*
		Chabertia ovina
		Cooperia spp.
		Haemonchus contortus
		H. placei
		Nematodirus spp.
		Neoascaris vitulorum
		Oesophagostomum radiatum
		O. venulosum
		Ostertagia spp.

Parasites Arranged by Host (Continued)

Group	Location	Species
		Strongyloides papillosus
		Trichostrongylus spp.
		Trichuris ovis
	Respiratory system	*Dictyocaulus viviparus*
	Skin and subcutaneous tissues	*Onchocerca cervicalis*
		Pelodera strongyloides
		Stephanofilaria stilesi
	Serous cavities	*Setaria cervi*
Cestodes	Digestive system	*Moniezia benedeni*
	Muscle and tendon	*Cysticercus bovis*
	Serous cavities	*Cysticercus tenuicollis*
	Liver	*Echinococcus granulosus*
Trematodes	Digestive system	*Paramphistomum* spp.
	Liver	*Dicrocoelium dendriticum*
		Fasciola hepatica
		Fascioloides magna
Arachnids	Skin and subcutaneous tissues	*Boophilus annulatus*
		Chorioptes bovis
		Demodex bovis
		Dermacentor albipictus
		D. variabilis
		Otobius megnini
		Psoroptes bovis
		Sarcoptes scabiei var. *bovis*
Insects	Urogenital system	*Eristalis tenax*
	Skin and subcutaneous tissues	*Bovicola bovis*
		Calliphora sp.
		Chrysops sp.
		Cochliomyia (Callitroga) hominivorax
		Haematobia irritans
		Haematopinus eurysternus
		Hypoderma bovis
		H. lineatum
		Linognathus vituli
		Lucilia sp.
		Musca autumnalis
		Phormia sp.
		Solenopotes capillatus
		Stomoxys calcitrans
		Tabanus spp.

Parasites Arranged by Host (Continued)

Group	Location	Species
	Sheep	
Protozoans	Digestive system	*Eimeria ninakohlyakimovae*
		E. ovina (arloingi)
		E. parva
	Circulatory system	*Trypanosoma melophagium*
	Muscle and tendon	*Sarcocystis* sp.
	Miscellaneous tissues	*Toxoplasma gondii*
Nematodes	Digestive system	*Bunostomum trigonocephalum*
		Chabertia ovina
		Cooperia spp.
		Gongylonema pulchrum
		Haemonchus contortus
		Nematodirus spp.
		Oesophagostomum columbianum
		Ostertagia circumcincta
		Strongyloides papillosus
		Trichostrongylus axei
		Trichostrongylus spp.
		Trichuris ovis
	Respiratory system	*Dictyocaulus filiaria*
		Muellerius capillaris
	Circulatory system	*Elaephora schneideri*
	Central nervous system	*Parelaphostrongylus tenuis*
Cestodes	Digestive system	*Moniezia expansa*
		Thysanosoma actinoides
	Respiratory system	*Echinococcus granulosus*
	Muscle and tendon	*Cysticercus ovis*
	Central nervous system	*Coenurus cerebralis*
	Liver	*Echinococcus granulosus*
Trematodes	Digestive system	*Cotylophoron* sp.
	Liver	*Dicrocoelium dendriticum*
		Fasciola hepatica
		Fascioloides magna
Arachnids	Skin and subcutaneous tissues	*Chorioptes ovis*
		Demodex ovis
		Dermacentor variabilis
		Otobius megnini
		Psorergates ovis
		Psoroptes ovis
Insects	Skin and subcutaneous tissues	*Bovicola ovis*
		Calliphora sp.

Parasites Arranged by Host (Continued)

Group	Location	Species
		Cochliomyia (Callitroga) hominivorax
		Linognathus pedalis
		Melophagus ovinus
		Oestrus ovis
		Phormia sp.

Pig

Group	Location	Species
Protozoans	Digestive system	*Balantidium coli*
		Eimeria debliecki
		Entamoeba coli
		E. histolytica
		E. suis
		Sarcocystis sp.
		Tritrichomonas suis
	Respiratory system	*Tritrichomonas suis*
	Muscle and tendon	*Sarcocystis* sp.
	Miscellaneous tissues	*Toxoplasma gondii*
Nematodes	Digestive system	*Ascaris suum*
		Ascarops strongylina
		Gongylonema pulchrum
		Hyostrongylus rubidus
		Oesophagostomum spp.
		Physocephalus sexaltus
		Stephanurus dentatus
		Strongyloides ransomi
		Trichinella spiralis
		Trichuris suis
	Respiratory system	*Metastrongylus* spp.
	Muscle and tendon	*Trichinella spiralis*
Cestodes	Respiratory system	*Echinococcus granulosus*
	Muscle and tendon	*Cysticercus cellulosae (T. solium)*
	Serous cavities	*Cysticercus tenuicollis*
	Liver	*Echinococcus granulosus*
Acanthocephalans	Digestive system	*Macracanthorhynchus hirudinaceus*
Arachnids	Skin and subcutaneous tissues	*Demodex phylloides*
		Dermacentor variabilis
		Sarcoptes scabiei var. *suis*
Insects	Skin and subcutaneous tissues	*Cochliomyia (Callitroga) hominivorax*
		Haematopinus suis

Parasites Arranged by Host (Continued)

Group	Location	Species
	Dog and Cat	
Protozoans	Digestive system	*Balantidium coli*
		Entamoeba coli
		E. histolytica
		Giardia canis
		G. cati
		Isospora bigemina
		I. canis
		I. felis
		I. rivolta
		Pentatrichomonas sp.
	Circulatory system	*Babesia canis*
		Leishmania donovani
		Trypanosoma cruzi
	Miscellaneous tissues	*Toxoplasma gondii*
Nematodes	Digestive system	*Ancylostoma braziliense*
		A. caninum
		A. tubaeforme
		Ollulanus tricuspis
		Physaloptera sp.
		Spirocerca lupi
		Strongyloides stercoralis var. *canis*
		Toxascaris leonina
		Toxocara canis
		T. cati (mystax)
		Trichuris vulpis
		Uncinaria stenocephala
	Respiratory system	*Aleurostrongylus abstrusus*
		Capillaria aerophila
		Crenosoma vulpis
		Filaroides hirthi
		F. milksi
		F. osleri
	Circulatory system	*Dipetalonema reconditum*
		Dirofilaria immitis
	Skin and subcutaneous tissues	*Dipetalonema reconditum*
		Dracunculus insignis
		Pelodera strongyloides
	Urogenital system	*Capillaria plica*
		Dioctophyma renale
	Eye	*Thelazia californiensis*
Cestodes	Digestive system	*Diphyllobothrium latum*
		Dipylidium caninum

Parasites Arranged by Host (Continued)

Group	Location	Species
		Echinococcus granulosus
		E. multilocularis
		Spirometra mansonoides
		Taenia hydatigena
		T. krabbei
		T. multiceps
		T. ovis
		T. pisiformis
		T. serialis
		T. taeniaformis
Trematodes	Digestive system	*Alaria canis*
		Nanophyetus salmincola
	Respiratory system	*Paragonimus kellicotti*
	Circulatory system	*Heterobilharzia americana*
	Liver	*Metorchis conjunctus*
		Platynosomum concinnum (fastosum)
Acanthocephalans	Digestive system	*Oncicola canis*
Arachnids	Respiratory system	*Pneumonyssoides caninum*
	Circulatory system	*Demodex folliculorum*
	Skin and subcutaneous tissues	*Cheyletiella parasitivorax*
		C. yasguri
		Demodex folliculorum
		Dermacentor variabilis
		Notoedres cati
		Otobius megnini
		Otodectes cynotis
		Rhipicephalus sanguineus
		Sarcoptes scabiei var. *canis*
		Trombicula spp.
Insects	Skin and subcutaneous tissues	*Cochliomyia (Callitroga) hominivorax*
		Ctenocephalides canis
		C. felis
		Cuterebra spp.
		Felicola subrostrata
		Heterodoxus sp.
		Linognathus setosus
		Pulex irritans
		Stomoxys calcitrans
		Trichodectes canis
		Wohlfahrtia vigil

Parasites Arranged by Host (Continued)

Group	Location	Species
Linguatulids	Respiratory system	*Linguatula serrata*

Chicken and Turkey

Group	Location	Species
Protozoans	Digestive system	*Eimeria acervulina*
		E. adenoeides
		E. brunetti
		E. hagani
		E. maxima
		E. meleagridis
		E. meleagrimitis
		E. mitis
		E. mivati
		E. necatrix
		E. praecox
		E. tenella
		Hexamita meleagridis
		Histomonas meleagridis
		Trichomonas gallinae
	Circulatory system	*Leucocytozoon smithi*
Nematodes	Digestive system	*Ascaridia dissimilis*
		A. galli
		Capillaria annulata
		C. contorta
		C. obsignata
		Cheilospirura hamulosa
		Heterakis gallinarum
		Tetrameres americana
	Respiratory system	*Syngamus trachea*
	Eye	*Oxyspirura mansoni*
Cestodes	Digestive system	*Davainea proglottina*
		Hymenolepis sp.
		Raillietina cesticellus
Trematodes	Digestive system	*Echinostoma revolutum*
	Urogenital system	*Prosthogonimus macrorchis*
	Skin and subcutaneous tissue	*Collyriclum faba*
Arachnids	Respiratory system	*Cytodites nudus*
	Skin and subcutaneous tissues	*Argas persicus*
		Cnemidocoptes mutans
		Dermanyssus gallinae
		Laminosioptes cysticola
		Ornithonyssus sylviarum
		Trombicula spp.

Parasites Arranged by Host (Continued)

Group	Location	Species
Insects	Skin and subcutaneous tissues	*Cimex lectularius*

Ducks and Geese

Group	Location	Species
Protozoans	Circulatory system	*Leucocytozoon simondi*
		Sarcocystis sp.
	Urogenital system	*Eimeria truncata*
Nematodes	Digestive system	*Amidostomum anseris*
		Capillaria contorta
		Tetrameres crami
Cestodes	Digestive system	*Hymenolepis* sp.
Trematodes	Digestive system	*Echinostoma revolutum*
	Urogenital system	*Prosthogonimus macrorchis*
	Skin and subcutaneous tissues	*Collyriclum faba*
Arachnids	Skin and subcutaneous tissues	*Argas persicus*
		Laminosioptes cysticola
		Trombicula spp.

Appendix C
Chemotherapeutic Agents

The agents mentioned in the handbook are commonly in use. Reference to commercial products or trade names is made with the understanding that no discrimination is intended and no endorsement by the author is implied. Mention of trade names does not constitute a guarantee or warranty of the products named. For specific, detailed information, the practitioner is referred to the directions of the manufacturer, especially with regard to dosage.

Chemotherapeutic Agents Commonly Used to Control Parasites

Parasites, grouped by host, are alphabetically arranged. Trade names, if included, are in parentheses following generic names of drugs. To convert kilograms into pounds, multiply the number of kilograms by 2.2; to convert pounds into kilograms, divide the number of pounds by 2.2. Abbreviations: (bw) = body weight; s/c = subcutaneous; I.V. = intravenous; I.M. = intramuscular.

Parasite	Drug	Dose and mode of administration
	Horse	
Anoplocephala	Niclosamide (Yomesan)	200-300 mg. per kg. (bw). Experimental.
Babesia	Phenamidine	9 mg. per kg. I.M. in multiple sites (as a 40% solution) on 2 consecutive days.
Gasterophilus	Dichlorvos Trichlorfon	4.5 gm. per 100 lb. (bw) as a paste. 18-36 gm. per 100 lb. (bw).
Habronema (cutaneous)	Phenol 5, oil of tar 10, and glycerine 85 parts.	Apply daily to lesion until healed.
Oxyuris	Thiabendazole Pyrantel Piperazine	2 gm. per 100 lb. (bw) in feed. 12.5 mg. per kg. (bw) drench. 5-7 gm. (base) per 100 lb. (bw) oral.

Chemotherapeutic Agents (Continued)

Parasite	Drug	Dose and mode of administration
Parascaris	Piperazine	5-7 gm. (base) per 100 lb. (bw) oral.
Probstmayria	Thiabendazole	2 gm. per 100 lb. (bw) in feed.
Strongyles, large and small	Thiabendazole	2 gm. per 100 lb. (bw) in feed.
	Phenothiazine (low level regimen)	2 gm. per adult. Daily in feed for 3 weeks of each month to reduce pasture contamination with eggs.
	Piperazine	5-7 gm. (base) per 100 lb. (bw).
Tritrichomonas	Iodochlorhydroxyquin	6-10 gm. per 1000 lb. (bw). Daily per os until improvement noted.
Trypanosoma	Antrycide	5 mg. per kg. (bw), 5% solution I.M.

Cattle

Parasite	Drug	Dose and mode of administration
Babesia	Phenamidine	9.0-13.5 mg. per kg. (bw) I.M.
	Berenil	3.5-5.0 mg. per kg. (bw) I.M.
	Acriflavine	200-400 ml. I.V. of 1:200-1:1000 solution.
Blowflies and screwworm	Smear E.Q. 335	Topical application.
	Coumaphos	0.125% aqueous spray or dip.
	Ronnel	0.5% as spray or dip.
Bunostomum	Levamisole	5.0-8.0 mg. per kg. (bw) per os. (Not for use in dairy cattle.)
Boophilus	Sodium arsenite	0.25% in final dip. External use only.
	Toxaphene	0.5% aqueous spray or dip (not on dairy cattle).
	Rotenone	0.01-0.1% as dip or spray.
	Coumaphos	0.25% dip (not for use on lactating cattle).
Coccidia	Amprolium	10 mg. kg. (bw) daily for 5 days in water.
Dictyocaulus	Levamisole	1.5-4.0 mg. per kg. (bw) parenterally.
Haemonchus	Levamisole	5-8 mg. per kg. (bw) oral.
Moniezia	Lead arsenate	0.5 gm., 40-50 lb. (bw). 1 gm., 50 lb. and over, per os.
	Niclosamide (Yomesan)	50 mg. per lb. (bw) per os.
	Dichlorophen	200-400 mg. per kg. (bw) per os.
Psoroptes	Lime sulfur	2.0-2.5% aqueous spray.
	Toxaphene	0.2-0.4% aqueous dip. Do not use on dairy cattle.
	Lindane (restricted use)	0.035% dip or spray. Do not use on milking cattle.

Chemotherapeutic Agents (Continued)

Parasite	Drug	Dose and mode of administration
Theileria	Chlortetracycline (For *Anaplasma* carriers)	For cattle, 5 mg. per lb. (bw) parenterally daily for 10 consecutive days.
Trichostrongyles	Tetramisole	15 mg. per kg. (bw) per os. (Dose not to exceed 4.5 gm.)
Tritrichomonas	Dimetridazole	50-60 mg. per kg. (bw). Daily, per os for 5 days.
	Acriflavine and Bovoflavin ointment	20 ml. of 1:1000 solution of acriflavine injected into urethra followed by application of 0.5% bovoflavin ointment topically.

Sheep

Parasite	Drug	Dose and mode of administration
Blowflies and screwworm	E. Q. 335	Topical application.
Bunostomum	Tetramisole	15 mg. per kg. (bw) drench.
Dicrocoelium	Thiabendazole	200-300 mg. per kg. (bw) drench.
Dictyocaulus	Levamisole	7.5 mg. per kg. (bw) s/c.
Haemonchus	Tetramisole	15 mg. per kg. (bw) oral. Not to exceed 600 mg. per dose.
Melophagus	Coumaphos Malathion	0.125% aqueous solution as spray or dip. 4-5% dust. Repeat at 2-3 week interval.
Moniezia	Lead arsenate	0.5 gm., 40-50 lb. (bw). 1.0 gm., 50 lb. or more per os.
	Niclosamide (Yomesan)	50 mg. per lb. (bw) per os.
	Dichlorophen	200-400 mg. per kg. (bw) per os.
Muellerius	Emetine hydrochloride	3 mg. per kg. I.M. as 1% solution of hydrochloride. 2-3 doses at 48 hr. intervals.
Oesophagostomum	Phenothiazine Thiabendazole Tetramisole	25 gm. 60 lb. or over. 44-88 mg. kg. (bw) per os. 15 mg. per kg. (bw) per os. Dose not to exceed 600 mg.
Psoroptes	Lime sulfur Toxaphene Lindane (restricted use)	2.0-2.5% aqueous spray. 0.2-0.4% aqueous spray or dip. 0.035% dip or spray. Do not use on milking cattle.
Trichostrongyles	Levamisole	7.5 mg. per kg. (bw) per os.

Chemotherapeutic Agents (Continued)

Parasite	Drug	Dose and mode of administration
	Pig	
Ascaris	Tetramisole	15 mg. per kg. (bw) in feed.
Haematopinus	Coumaphos	0.06% spray.
	Toxaphene	0.5% spray.
Hyostrongylus	Dichlorvos	15-40 mg. per kg. (bw) in feed.
	Tetramisole	15 mg. per kg. (bw) in feed).
Metastrongylus	Tetramisole	15 mg. per kg. (bw) in feed.
	Levamisole	3.6 mg. per lb. (bw) in feed.
Oesophagostomum	Thiabendazole	100 mg. per kg. (bw) in feed.
	Phenothiazine	10 gm. per 100 lb. (bw).
Sarcoptes	Lime sulfur	2.0-2.5% spray.
	Chlordane	1.0% aqueous spray or dip.
	Malathion	0.6% spray.
Strongyloides	Thiabendazole	50 mg. per kg. (bw) in feed. 30-40 mg. per lb. (bw) paste formuation.
Trichuris	Dichlorvos	15-40 mg. per kg. (bw) in feed.
	Dog	
Ancylostoma	Disophenol (DNP)	4.5 mg. per lb. (bw) s/c.
	Thenium closylate (Canopar)	500 mg. per 10 lb. (bw) or more oral.
	Dichlorvos	27 mg. per lb. (bw) per os.
Dipylidium	Niclosamide (Yomesan)	500 mg. per 7 lb. (bw) tablets.
	Bunamidine (Scolaban)	25 mg. per kg. (bw) in feed. 2 doses at 4-day interval.
Dirofilaria	Thiacetarsamide (caparsolate sodium)	0.1 ml. per lb. (bw) I.V. twice a day for 2 days.
D. immitis (microfilariae)	Dithiazinine	2.0 mg. per lb. (bw) oral. Daily for 7 days.
Echinococcus	Bunamidine (Scolaban)	25-50 mg. per kg. (bw) in food.
Entamoeba	Bismuth glycolylarsanilate (Milibis)	100 mg. per lb. (bw). Daily for 5 days per os.
	Metronidazole (Flagyl)	50 mg. per kg. (bw). Daily for 5 days per os.
Filaroides	Levamisole	7.5 mg. per kg. (bw) oral.
Giardia	Metronidazole (Flagyl)	50 mg. per kg. (bw) daily for 5 days per os.

Chemotherapeutic Agents (Continued)

Parasite	Drug	Dose and mode of administration
	Atabrine	20 mg. per kg. (bw) daily for 6 days per os.
	Bismuth glycolylarsanilate (Milibis)	100 mg./lb. (bw), per os daily for 5 days.
Isospora *Eimeria*	Sulfonamides, enteric	25 mg. per lb. (bw) per os. Treat daily until signs alleviated.
Otodectes	Canex	1 part Canex with 3 parts mineral oil topically. Repeat each 5-7 days as indicated.
	Rotenone	.03% in oil topically.
Sarcoptes	Benzyl benzoate	Use every 2-3 days topically. Not more than 7 treatments without professional evaluation.
	Chlordane	0.5% dip. Topically.
Taenia	Bunamidine (Scolaban)	25 mg. per kg. (bw) in feed. 2 doses at 4-day interval.
	Niclosamide (Yomesan)	500 mg. per 7 lb. (bw) oral.
	Nemural	18 mg. per 8 lb. (bw) oral.
Toxascaris and *Toxocara*	Piperazine	20-30 mg. per lb. (bw) oral.
	Dichlorvos	27 mg. per 2 lb. (bw) oral.
	Diethylcarbamazine	20-30 mg. per lb. (bw) oral.
	Butyl chloride	1 ml. per 5 lb. (bw) oral.
Toxoplasma	Pyrimethamine plus sulfadiazine (Daraprim)	1 mg. per lb. (bw) for 3 days, then 0.5 mg. per lb. for 3 days oral.
Trichuris	Phthalofyne (Whipcide)	100 mg. per lb. (bw) oral.
	Dichlorvos	27 mg. per 2 lbs. (bw)
	Bismuth glycolylarsanilate (Milibis)	100 mg. per lb. (bw) per os daily for 5 days.
Poultry		
Amidostomum	Tetramisole	40 mg. per kg. (bw) in feed or water.
	Pyrantel tartrate	100 mg. per kg. (bw) in feed.
Ascaridia	Tetramisole	40-50 mg. per kg. (bw) in feed or capsule.
Capillaria	Tetramisole	40-50 mg. per kg. (bw) in feed or capsule.
Heterakis	Tetramisole	40-50 mg. per kg. (bw) in feed or capsule.
Hymenolepis	Dibutyl tin dilaurate	125 mg. per kg. (bw) in feed.
Leucocytozoon	Clopidol (For turkeys)	0.025% in feed.
Ornithonyssus	Carbaryl (Sevin)	40% fogging spray.

Chemotherapeutic Agents (Continued)

Parasite	Drug	Dose and mode of administration
Raillietina	Niclosamide (Yomesan)	50 mg. per kg. (bw) in feed.
Syngamus	Thiabendazole	0.1% in feed for 2 weeks.

Selected references:

Allen, L. J., J. R. Marshall, L. A. Nall, M. C. Thomas, and H. E. Jordan. 1976. Compendium of chemotherapeutic agents for parasitic protozoa and helminths of dogs and cats. *Vet. Med. Small Anim. Clin.* 71:1083-88.

Gibson, T. E. 1975. *Veterinary Anthelmintic Medication*, 3rd Edition, Commonwealth Agr. Bureau, Tech. Comm. No. 33.

Rossoff, J. S. 1974. *Handbook of Veterinary Drugs.* New York: Springer.

GLOSSARY

Glossary

Acanthocephalan: A nematodelike worm that has a spiny proboscis and no alimentary canal.

Acetabulum: An organ of attachment, usually on the anterior third of the ventral surface of many flukes. It is also called the ventral sucker.

Adanal shields: Paired, sclerotized structures on the ventral surface of male ticks of the genera *Boophilus*, *Rhipicephalus*, and *Hyalomma*.

Alae: Longitudinal ridges or flanges of cuticle on the lateral surfaces of some nematodes. They may be cervical or caudal.

Anterior station: Anterior part of the alimentary tract of a vector.

Arachnid: A member of the class Arachnida, which includes such arthropods as ticks, mites, spiders, and scorpions.

Autoinfection: An infection in which the source of reexposure for a host is the host itself.

Axostyle: A rodlike organelle that functions as an internal, structural support in certain protozoans, especially intestinal and vaginal flagellates.

Basis capitulum: In hard ticks the anterior movable portion that bears the mouth parts.

Bothria: Slitlike grooves on the scolex of pseudophyllidean tapeworms.

Bursa: An umbrellalike expansion of the cuticle at the posterior end of the male in all species of the order Strongyloidea.

Cercaria: A free-living larval trematode that develops from a sporocyst or redia in a snail host.

Cestode: A common name applied to the group of flatworms also known as tapeworms.

Cilia: Minute, hairlike organelles of locomotion in protozoans of the class Ciliata.

Coenurus *(Multiceps):* A larva that develops from a hexacanth embryo. The larva consists of a fluid-filled bladder, and numerous scolices develop on its inner wall.

Coracidium: A ciliated, free-swimming larva that hatches from the egg of a pseudophyllidean cestode.

Cyst: An immobile, protozoan stage that has a resistant protective layer and is often adapted for transmission to a new host.

Cysticercoid: A minute larval tapeworm resembling a cysticercus. However, the small bladder contains little or no fluid and one scolex. This form is usually found in an invertebrate.

Cysticercus: A larval stage of a taeniod tapeworm consisting of a bladderlike form containing fluid and a single scolex.

Definitive or primary host: A host that harbors the adult or sexually mature stages of the parasite.

Ectoparasite: A parasite that lives on the body surface of its host.

Embryophore: A membrane or thickened wall around the hexacanth embryo of tapeworms. It usually forms the inner portion of the egg shell.

Endogenous: Originating or produced within the organism.

Endoparasite: A parasite that lives within the body of its host.

Erratic parasite: A parasite that migrates to a location that is not its usual habitat.

Facultative parasite: An organism capable of either a free-living or a parasitic existence.

Festoon: Rectangular chitinous structures, separated by grooves and located on the posterior border of most genera of hard ticks.

Flagellate: A protozoan that has at least one whiplike flagellum as the organ of locomotion.

Gametocyte (Gamont): A cell capable of dividing to produce gametes.

Goblets: Small structures of various shapes in the spiracular plates of arthropods.

Habitat: The natural abode of an organism.

Helminth: A general term applied to the parasitic worms.

Hexacanth (Onchosphere): A 6-hooked embryo that hatches from the egg of tapeworms.

Host: An organism that harbors a parasite.

Hydatid *(Echinococcus):* A larval, tapeworm cyst developing from a hexacanth embryo. Many scolices may develop inside the cyst, and daughter cysts or brood capsules may develop there as well.

Incidental parasite: One that becomes established in an organism in which it does not ordinarily live.

Inornate tick: A tick in which the coloration of the scutum is not patterned.

Intermediate host: One that harbors the larval or asexual stages of a parasite. The 1st intermediate host is parasitized by the immature stages of the parasite. The 2nd intermediate host harbors an immature parasitic stage that has left the 1st intermediate host. If more than one intermediate host is required, the 1st is usually an invertebrate.

Intermittent parasite: One that makes brief visits to its host to obtain food and other benefits.

Interproglottid glands: A continuous row of small glands along the posterior border of the mature segment in *Moniezia* spp.

Lappet: A small, tablike structure behind the suckers of *Anoplocephala perfoliata.*

Leaf crown: Leaflike, cuticular structures around the anterior margin of the buccal capsule of certain nematodes.

Linguatulid: A member of the class Pentastomida commonly called tongueworms, an arthropod group allied to the mites.

Merozoite: A motile, infective stage of a sporozoan protozoan that results from schizogony or a similar type of asexual reproduction. It is also known as a zoite.

Metacercaria: An encysted, infective stage of a trematode. It is usually found in fish or crustacean tissues or on aquatic or semiaquatic vegetation.

Metamorphosis (complete): In some insects, development in which the larva is transformed into a pupa before emerging as an adult. The external form of the adult is entirely different from the form of the larva or pupa.

Miracidium: A free-swimming, 1st-stage larva of a trematode. This ciliated form penetrates the body of a snail.

Myiasis: The invasion of tissues or body cavities by the larvae of dipterous insects.

Nematode: A common name given to roundworms of the class Nematoda.

Onchosphere: See Hexacanth.

Operculum: A cap or lid that covers the opening through which the embryo of certain flukes and tapeworms escapes at hatching.

Ornate tick: A hard tick in which a blotchy color pattern is superimposed on the base color of the scutum.

Parasitosis: An infection or infestation in which the parasite injures its host causing disease signs or lesions and apparent illness.

Paratenic host: An intermediate or transfer host not essential to the completion of the parasite's life cycle.

Permanent parasite: One that is parasitic throughout its entire life history.

Plerocercoid: A wormlike larval tapeworm with an invaginated scolex. It is usually found in the flesh of a fish, its intermediate host.

Posterior station: Posterior part of the alimentary tract of a vector.

Prepatent period: The period between entry of an infective stage into the definitive or final host and the time at which a subsequent stage of the parasite within the host can be demonstrated.

Procercoid: A larval stage of a tapeworm in the body cavity of a crustacean, the 1st intermediate host.

Pseudoparasite: Any object resembling or mistaken for a parasite.

Ray: Elongated stalks or fingerlike processes of modified caudal papillae that support the bursal lobes.

Redia: A saclike larval trematode which develops in the body of a snail host. The muscular larva has both mouth and gut.

Rhabditiform larva: A nematode larva with a muscular, bulbed esophagus.

Rostellum: The anterior part of the scolex of certain tapeworms. It may be armed or unarmed depending on species.

Schizogony: Asexual reproduction of certain protozoans by multiple fission.

Schizont: A sporozoan trophozoite that reproduces by schizogony.

Scolex: The attachment organ at the cephalic end of a tapeworm.

Scutum (shield): A sclerotized dorsal plate posterior to the capitulum of hard ticks.

Sparganum: The plerocercoid larva of pseudophyllidian tapeworms of the genus *Spirometra*.

Spiracle: An opening to the tracheal system of many arthropods.

Sporocyst: A saclike larval fluke that develops in the body of its intermediate host, usually a snail. It produces either rediae or more sporocysts.

Sporozoite: A minute protozoan body resulting from the multiple division of the zygote.

Strobilia: A chain of segments comprising the bulk of the body of adult tapeworms.

Transovarian transmission: Passage of a microorganism into the egg or embryo within the body of an infected female host. An infection is thus transferred from mother to offspring.

Transport host: An organism that carries a parasite to another host. The parasite undergoes no development in the transport host.

Trans-stadial transmission: Passage of a microorganism from one stage of a host to another, through one or more molts. Usually used to refer to such transmission in an arthropod host.

Trematode: A common name for flatworms of the class Trematoda, also called flukes.

Trophozoite: The vegetative, motile stage of a protozoan parasite.

Viviparous: The production of active, living young by the female. No egg-laying occurs.

Xenodiagnosis: A method of diagnosis in which a natural, uninfected vector is fed on a suspected definitive host and later examined for parasites.

INDEX

Index